The Elephant in the Room: Practical Advice When the Diagnosis is Cancer

The Elephant in the Room: Practical Advice When the Diagnosis is Cancer

iUniverse, Inc.
Bloomington

THE ELEPHANT IN THE ROOM
PRACTICAL ADVICE WHEN THE DIAGNOSIS IS CANCER

Copyright © 2011 by Bob Riter.

All rights reserved. No part of this book may be used or reproduced by any means, graphic, electronic, or mechanical, including photocopying, recording, taping or by any information storage retrieval system without the written permission of the publisher except in the case of brief quotations embodied in critical articles and reviews.

The information, ideas, and suggestions in this book are not intended as a substitute for professional medical advice. Before following any suggestions contained in this book, you should consult your personal physician. Neither the author nor the publisher shall be liable or responsible for any loss or damage allegedly arising as a consequence of your use or application of any information or suggestions in this book.

iUniverse books may be ordered through booksellers or by contacting:

iUniverse
1663 Liberty Drive
Bloomington, IN 47403
www.iuniverse.com
1-800-Authors (1-800-288-4677)

Because of the dynamic nature of the Internet, any web addresses or links contained in this book may have changed since publication and may no longer be valid. The views expressed in this work are solely those of the author and do not necessarily reflect the views of the publisher, and the publisher hereby disclaims any responsibility for them.

Any people depicted in stock imagery provided by Thinkstock are models, and such images are being used for illustrative purposes only.
Certain stock imagery © Thinkstock.

ISBN: 978-1-4620-4658-4 (sc)
ISBN: 978-1-4620-4659-1 (hc)
ISBN: 978-1-4620-4660-7 (ebk)

Printed in the United States of America

iUniverse rev. date: 08/25/2011

Table of Contents

Introduction ix
Acknowledgments xi
Foreword xiii

Just Diagnosed 1
   Advice for those Newly Diagnosed 3
   Cancer and Positive Thinking 5
   It's OK to Ask Your Doctor These Questions 7
   How Old is too Old to Treat Cancer? 10
   Second Opinions 12
   If Your Mom has Cancer 14
   Good Cancers and Bad Cancers 16
   Telling the Kids 18
   Telling the Parents 20
   What to Say—and Not Say 22
   When a Loved One Has Cancer 24
   Thoughts and Prayer Tree 26

During Treatment 29
   Keeping Yourself in Balance 31
   Non-Traditional Cancer Therapies 34
   Doctor-Patient Interactions 37
   A Better Phrase than Staying Strong 40
   Advocating for a Loved One 42
   Groundhog Friends 44
   Helping from a Distance 46
   Helping Those We Don't Like 48
   Practical Ways to Help 50
   Chemobrain 52
   More than Tired 54

Understanding Friends with Cancer 56
　　Visiting Those in the Hospital 58
　　Single with Cancer 60
　　Cancer as a Marathon 62
　　Holiday Gifts 64
　　Holiday Gifts for those with Serious Illness 66
　　When a Partner is in Denial 68

After Treatment 71
　　The After-Treatment Blahs 73
　　When Loved Ones Complete Treatment 75
　　Survivor's Guilt 77
　　Post-Cancer Relationships 79
　　Donating Blood and Organs 81
　　Survivors Can Help the Newly Diagnosed 83
　　Cancer as a Chronic Disease 85
　　Beginning to talk about Hospice 87

Personal Reflections and Random Essays EssaysEssays 89
　　My Cancer Experience 91
　　Don't Ask about My Battle 93
　　Surprising Facts about Cancer 95
　　Uncertainty and Commitments 97
　　The Ugly Stepsister of Cancer 99
　　Cancer and the Nature of Hope 101
　　I have cancer. What's new with you? 103
　　My Cancer Sucks Button 105
　　Small Acts of Heroism 107
　　The Uncertainty of Cancer 109
　　The Difficult Transitions of Cancer 111
　　The Good That Emerged 113
　　The Look People Give You 115
　　Stepping Up for Neighbors 117
　　New Year's Wishes 119

Our Cancer Professionals 121
New Nurses and Cancer Patients 123
Doing What I Do 125

Introduction

It can be awkward talking with a friend or loved one who has been diagnosed with cancer. What should you say? What should you *not* say?

If you have cancer, you may wonder if it's OK to ask your physician the questions you most want to ask.

Even health professionals sometimes feel self-conscious when talking with their patients who have cancer.

The purpose of this book is to help people have conversations about cancer. We don't need to tiptoe around the elephant in the room.

I didn't give much thought to cancer until I was diagnosed with breast cancer in 1996. In hindsight, being a male with breast cancer gave me a unique vantage point from which to see cancer from a variety of perspectives. I was a guy with what's typically a woman's cancer, so I had access to and became comfortable with women and men with all kinds of cancers. And while breast cancer is common, male breast cancer is rare, so I got to experience both ends of the *rare cancer — common cancer* continuum.

For the past eleven years, I've had the privilege of working at the Cancer Resource Center of the Finger Lakes (originally known as the Ithaca Breast Cancer Alliance). The best part of my job is talking with people who are somehow affected by cancer. The columns in this book are largely based on those conversations.

Acknowledgments

Thanks to Sue Riter, Donna Heilweil, Kerry Quinn, Marguerite Sterling, Kat Lynch, Bev Johnson, and Irene Kolberg who routinely provided feedback on early drafts of my columns.

Thanks to the *Ithaca Journal* and its editor, Bruce Estes, for taking a chance on a regular column about living with cancer. And thank you to the *Ithaca Journal* and Gannett for granting permission for those columns to be compiled into this book.

Thanks to Andrea Kutsko Staffeld for her delightful illustrations that are used throughout the book.

Thanks to Cindie Frost for her layout expertise.

Thanks to Sue Riter for editing the manuscript.

Thanks to the Social Service League of Ithaca for donating the seed money required to make this book a reality.

Thanks to the staff of the Cancer Resource Center—Jyl Dowd, Sharon Kaplan, and Kerry Quinn—for sharing the joys and challenges of this work with me.

Thanks to the many volunteers of the Cancer Resource Center who constantly give of their time and of their hearts.

And special thanks to Sandy Meek True whose initiative and positive energy made this book happen.

Foreword

When I was five my mother found a lump in her breast. She was ordered to the hospital by her physician for a biopsy. She awoke a few hours later; her left breast was gone. She was left with severe lymphedema and a sense of shame about her body that stayed with her for the remaining 10 years of her life, when the disease returned to attack the other breast and her lungs. I remember her saying "I'm not supposed to know, but I have cancer." She died at the age of 46.

That story has shaped my life, influenced career choices, sensitized me to the struggle of not only patients but families as they cope with serious illness. Certainly medicine has changed since her death in 1954. Patients are now required to give permission for surgery, treatment modalities have become infinitely more sophisticated, and the important role of family and friends has been accepted. Many types of cancer have come to be viewed as chronic illness rather than terminal disease. Cancer is not viewed as if it were the plague, as Susan Sontag so aptly describes in her groundbreaking work, *Illness as Metaphor*. Yet the word cancer, when pronounced in a doctor's office, still brings with it a sense of shock, fear and confusion.

I have followed Bob Riter's career with interest and admiration. I first got to know him when we both served on the Board of Directors of ICaN, a volunteer organization that provided support to cancer patients. Bob was at that time on the staff of what was then the Ithaca Breast Cancer Alliance (IBCA). As he described the information and services IBCA offered to patients and their loved ones, we discussed how important it was to find a way to expand this care to people with all types of cancer. A few years later, the Board of IBCA decided to become the Cancer Resource Center of the Finger Lakes, of which Bob is now Executive Director. This decision has touched the lives of thousands of men, women and children in our community.

The columns collected in this immensely useful book come out of both Bob's personal experience with cancer and his years of counseling patients and those who support them. There is a practical wisdom to the way Bob addresses the issues: how to talk to your doctor, make informed medical decisions, cope with post-treatment anxiety, be most helpful to someone recently diagnosed or undergoing treatment. The columns contain ideas for maximizing comfort, both physical and emotional. And they reflect some of the struggles and victories of living with this potentially life-threatening illness. The writing is characterized by empathy grounded in realism; there is no false reassurance, nor is there deep pessimism. Instead there is a gentle reminder of the value of every day of our lives, and a reminder to people with cancer that they are not alone.

Nina Miller
Retired Executive Director,
Hospicare & Palliative Care Services
of Tompkins County

Just Diagnosed

Advice for those Newly Diagnosed

The first few days following a cancer diagnosis are like riding on top of a speeding train. You're hanging on for dear life and can't quite see what's ahead. Although every situation is somewhat different, this is what I generally suggest:

Focus on one step at a time. If you're having a biopsy next week, focus on that biopsy and don't let your mind wander to what might happen next. It's easy to overwhelm yourself with thousands of "what if" questions.

Family members, friends, and complete strangers will give you advice. Be wary if they say, "You should do . . ." Though well-intentioned, they don't know what's best for you. You do.

Remember that cancer treatments change rapidly. The treatment that was standard three years ago may not be standard today. What you hear from people treated in the past is usually out of date.

We often talk about cancer as a single disease, but there are over two hundred types of cancer. Don't assume that what you hear about one type of cancer holds true for other cancers as well.

Survival statistics are averages. They can be helpful if you want a general idea of what will happen, on average, to a large group of people with your disease, but they can't predict what will happen to you.

Don't hesitate to get a second opinion if you think it might be helpful. Your doctor won't mind. (If your doctor does mind, you should get another doctor.)

A new cancer diagnosis is rarely a medical emergency. You generally have several days or even weeks to explore your options. (Some situations do require immediate attention—ask your doctor how long it's safe to wait before beginning treatment.)

Don't begin a radical "cancer curing" diet or major lifestyle change during treatment. Just eat sensibly and nutritiously, exercise moderately, and get plenty of rest. You can make whatever lifestyle and diet changes you want after treatment is over.

Medications that control side effects have improved tremendously, but not every medication works equally well for each person. Don't suffer in silence. Tell your doctor when you feel lousy. Other drugs may work better for you.

Nearly everyone undergoing cancer treatment experiences fatigue. It's probably the most common and least publicized side effect. Conserve your energy for activities that are most important to you.

Recovery is not a straight line. You'll feel better one day; then you'll feel worse; then you'll feel better. Don't be discouraged by the down days.

The end of treatment is not necessarily a time of celebration. For many people, it's the most difficult time because you want to get back to your old routine, but you still feel tired and blah. Be patient with yourself.

Don't blame yourself for your cancer. It's usually impossible to say why an individual got cancer. And no one—no one—deserves cancer.

Cancer and Positive Thinking

Whenever someone is diagnosed with cancer, people feel compelled to say, "You gotta stay positive!" (This is usually said with an enthusiastic pump of the arm.)

I'm a pretty positive guy and I'm all in favor of positive thinking, but I cringe whenever I hear those words.

First of all, telling someone to be positive has never transformed anyone into actually being positive. I've yet to hear someone respond, "You're absolutely right. I've never thought about being positive, but now that you mention it, I see the wisdom in it. I will become positive and change my outlook on life." That just doesn't happen, at least not in my world.

My real concern is for people with cancer who may blame themselves for not being positive enough. How does one make sense of a recurrence if positive thinking is supposed to help? I hope no one sees their recurrence as the result of not thinking enough positive thoughts. People with cancer don't need another reason to beat themselves up.

Don't get me wrong—I think it's great to have a positive attitude when dealing with cancer. I did, and I'm sure it was helpful in my recovery.

If my cancer returns, I will again be positive. If there's only a five percent chance of survival, I figure that I'm going to be in that five percent.

But attitude is largely a function of personality, and you are who you are. Positive people enjoy having other positive people and positive energy around them. People who aren't so positive don't necessarily want or benefit from cheerleaders in the room.

And even the sunniest, most positive people will have down days when dealing with cancer. It's a scary, life-changing event and filled with uncertainty. Rather than telling them to be positive, acknowledge and share in their sadness on those days. Doing so makes an honest connection.

Cancer is no different than every other aspect of life. We need to face it in our own way and on our own terms.

And our dearest friends and family members will accept those terms, and support us and love us no matter what.

It's OK to Ask Your Doctor These Questions

People often leave their doctor's offices irritated with themselves for not asking what they wanted to ask. Sometimes they simply forget to ask. (I encourage people to bring a list.) On other occasions, though, people aren't sure if it's OK to ask certain questions. Sometimes the questions that people hesitate to ask are the ones that they're most concerned about. These are some of those questions:

How much will this cost? Being treated for cancer can be incredibly expensive. In general, people want to know what they'll have to pay out of their own pocket. Someone in the medical office should be able to give you a reasonable estimate of what your insurance will pay and what will be your responsibility.

Is there a less expensive alternative? We all want the best possible care, and physicians want us to have that care. But say, for example, that you have no health insurance at all and you're paying from your life savings. The newest and best drug for your cancer might cost $50,000 for a course of treatment. An older generation drug might be ninety-five percent as effective as the newest drug, but cost only $1,000. Is that a reasonable trade-off? It's an individual decision, but it's fair to ask the question.

What's the likely benefit from a proposed treatment? Cancer treatment is about improving your odds of preventing a recurrence and extending your life. You can ask, "How much will this chemotherapy/radiation/surgery improve my odds of preventing a recurrence?" Sometimes the likely benefit is huge, sometimes the benefit is small, and sometimes it's uncertain.

Do I need all of the proposed treatments? Sometimes the suggested treatment includes radiation AND chemotherapy AND hormonal treatment, etc. You can ask, "If I get chemotherapy, what's the added benefit of radiation? Or, if I get radiation therapy, what's the added benefit of chemotherapy?" We don't always have clear evidence, but these are reasonable questions to ask.

How long can I wait before beginning treatment? Some cancers require that treatment begin quickly. Other cancers are slow moving and treatment can safely wait for many weeks. You can quite possibly spend time exploring other options or just going ahead with that long-planned vacation.

How long am I likely to live? Some people want to know their prognosis and others don't. Doctor can't predict precisely how long you will live, but they can give you a general idea of what's typical for people with your condition. It's OK to ask. And it's OK not to ask.

Is hospice a reasonable option? As more and more treatments become available to treat advanced cancers, there's almost always something to try when the current treatment stops working. At some point, many people wonder if it's worth pursuing those additional treatments. You can ask your doctor if hospice is a reasonable option to consider.

Can you repeat that? People usually miss a good deal of what their doctor tells them, especially if it's a stressful time. (Hearing that you have cancer is always stressful.) Don't be afraid to ask a doctor to repeat something.

Many of these questions don't have simple answers. People with cancer often have to make decisions with incomplete information. No one knows for certain how an individual will respond to a particular treatment or what the future might hold. Sometimes the answer to these questions will be, "I don't know" or "there's no data on that." But asking questions is always OK.

How Old is too Old to Treat Cancer?

The older you are, the more likely it is that you'll be diagnosed with cancer. The average age at diagnosis is now 66 and it's increasingly common for people in their late 80s and even older to consider cancer treatment.

Is this a good thing?

I think it's great when an 85-year-old says, "I want to aggressively treat my cancer. Give me chemo, give me whatever."

But I cringe when the relatives of an 85-year-old say, "We want to aggressively treat our father's cancer. Give him chemo, give him whatever."

The distinction, of course, is in who's making the request.

Treatment decisions are based on the likely benefits (e.g., extending one's life) and the likely costs (e.g., unpleasant side effects) of that treatment. Neither is known with certainty because there is so much individual variation, but doctors can provide some general guidance. They might say, "This treatment is relatively easy to tolerate and may extend your life for a few months, but no one knows for sure."

It's then up to the patient to decide if the treatment is worth pursuing. I'm very wary if I sense the family is more interested in aggressive treatment than is the patient. This is sometimes communicated quite subtly, "Oh Dad. I don't know if Mom can manage without you."

I also think some people pursue aggressive treatment because they "don't want to disappoint their doctors." Please don't worry about disappointing your doctors. They almost always have one more drug to try, and they're trained to keep trying.

I said I love it when an 85-year-old wants to aggressively treat his cancer. I also love it when an 85-year-old says, "I've had a good life and now I want to focus on the quality of my remaining life. Don't give me drugs to extend my life if those drugs will make me feel worse."

There may be less aggressive treatment options worth considering. In the United States, we tend to assume that the most aggressive treatment is always the "best" treatment. This isn't always the case, especially when factoring in quality of life. Perhaps there's another chemotherapy protocol that's easier to tolerate and still beneficial.

And be cautious if deciding on no additional treatment. Sometimes people say, "No more treatment" when they mean to say, "No more *life-extending* treatment." Radiation therapy is often given to reduce pain. Even some surgical procedures and chemotherapy treatments are designed not to extend life, but to provide comfort. Keep these options open.

Physicians and family members should also realize that age is not a good predictor of what others might decide. A few decades ago, some doctors automatically performed mastectomies on older patients with breast cancer (rather than considering less extensive surgery) because they assumed that older women wouldn't mind losing a breast. A word of advice I freely share with my readers: never, ever make assumptions about anyone else's body parts.

Second Opinions

People diagnosed with cancer sometimes ask me if their doctor will take offense if they get a second opinion.

The answer is no. Nearly all doctors today are receptive to patients getting second opinions. (And if you have one of those rare doctors that does take offense, you should seriously consider getting a new doctor.)

Your doctors want you to be comfortable with the treatment decisions that are made. And they want you to feel comfortable with them as individuals. Treating cancer is often a life-long partnership between the two of you.

Second opinions are especially beneficial when there are significantly different treatment options available. For example, surgery, radiation therapy, and "watchful waiting" are often reasonable options to consider for the treatment of prostate cancer. Talking with different types of physicians is often helpful.

Here are a few practical suggestions:

- It's entirely appropriate to ask your doctor for a recommendation as to where to go for a second opinion. This is especially true for rare cancers. You'll want a second opinion from someone who sees that particular type of cancer on a regular basis. In addition, your doctor's office can help arrange the appointment and send a copy of your medical records for you.

- You should ask your doctor how long you can safely wait before beginning treatment. Some cancers are relatively slow moving and a month's delay in beginning treatment won't make any difference. Other cancers are more aggressive and treatment should begin quickly. It's sometimes reasonable to obtain a second opinion even after treatment has started.

You should generally obtain the second opinion from a physician who is not associated with your first physician. Physicians who work together tend to share similar philosophies and practice patterns.

You may be able to obtain a second opinion without leaving town by arranging a telephone consultation. Major cancer centers are often able to provide opinions based on your medical records.

We usually think of second opinions in terms of treatment decisions, but it's also possible to request a second opinion on the pathology itself. That is, your slides can be sent to another institution for a different pathologist to review.

What should you do if your second opinion differs from the original recommendation? You can ask the two doctors to talk with each other to see if they can reach a consensus. You can seek a third opinion. Another option I recommend is to meet with your family doctor. He or she can often explain the options, place them in context, and help you reach a decision.

If Your Mom has Cancer

I sometimes hear from middle-aged friends who tell me that their mother (or father) was just diagnosed with cancer. They then launch into their plans for her treatment.

This is when I ask, "What does your mom want?"

This question is usually met by a four- or five-second pause, followed by a hesitant, "What do you mean?"

"I mean, what does your mom want? Have you asked her?"

You'd be surprised how often mom hasn't been asked.

In some cases, adult children want mom to have the most aggressive treatment possible, even if that treatment is likely to extend her life for only a few months and at the cost of making her miserable.

In other cases, children want to take their mother across the country to the world's expert on her disease when she would be more comfortable staying with the doctors who know her and have treated her for many years.

Sometimes the most aggressive therapy is the best approach, and sometimes it does make sense to travel to see the world's expert. But, please, don't make assumptions about what your mother wants. Ask her.

It's often helpful to involve your mother's primary care physician in the decision-making process. The specialists involved in your mother's care will focus on what *can* be done. The primary care physician can help your mother sort through what *should* be done, based on her overall condition, her wishes, and a host of other factors.

What's most important for a daughter or son in dealing with a mother's cancer is simply to be present for her. Be available when she wants to talk and support her in the choices she makes. This is hard for many of us because we're accustomed to fixing things. We tend to focus too much on the fix and not enough on the person.

Health care providers will naturally focus on your mother's cancer. As a family member, you have the opportunity and privilege of focusing on her as a person. It's the best gift you'll ever give her.

Good Cancers and Bad Cancers

I routinely talk with people who have just been diagnosed with cancer. They're struggling with treatment decisions and the realization that life is suddenly different.

I also talk with people with advanced cancer who are coming to terms with a poor prognosis and the realization that, in all likelihood, they will die prematurely because of that cancer.

It is particularly devastating to receive both rounds of bad news at once—that you have cancer and that a cure is unlikely.

In the regular world, all cancer is bad, but in oncology offices, there are good cancers and there are bad cancers. I realize that "good cancer" sounds like an oxymoron, but cancer professionals often think in those terms. Good cancers are generally curable.

Of course, if it's your cancer, it's never a "good cancer," a "garden variety cancer," or any other term that seemingly diminishes your fears or the disruption of your life.

Breast cancer and prostate cancer are the most common cancers (aside from skin cancer), and they're generally "good" cancers. People who receive these diagnoses undergo treatment and then return to their normal lives. In all likelihood, they will die many years later of something else.

But people who are diagnosed with the "bad" cancers often die from those cancers. New treatments are increasingly able to extend lives—often for many years—but a cure is the exception rather than the rule.

There are, however, survivors of even the worst diagnoses. I love meeting people who were treated for "bad" cancers years ago and are still going strong. There are no absolutes.

And many cancers fall somewhere in between being a good cancer and a bad cancer on the spectrum of cancer survivability. In some ways, people with these cancers have the most difficult time of all because statistics don't provide a clear roadmap for what's ahead.

I find that patients diagnosed with bad cancers often accept the news better than do their loved ones.

Patients generally accept the reality of the situation *and* maintain their sense of hope. Reality and hope aren't mutually exclusive. In fact, the patients who keep reality and hope in balance almost always seem to have an easier time—emotionally and physically—than those who lose that balance.

And loved ones who maintain a similar balance are the best companions for this difficult journey. Every patient with cancer has days of confidence and days of fear. Loved ones who listen and support every day are special treasures.

Telling the Kids

If you are diagnosed with cancer when you have young children, you're faced with what to share with them and how to share it.

It is important to realize that cancer affects the entire family and not just the person with cancer. As a member of that family, children have the right to be included.

Children can usually sense when something is wrong. And they will likely overhear the word "cancer" when you're talking with someone else. If you tell them the truth, they can focus on the reality rather than the even scarier things in their imagination.

When you talk with your children, it is important to use language they understand and to be sensitive to their concerns.

Here are a few suggestions:

> Children need to be assured of their own security. How will family life change as a result of what's happening? Who will pick them up from school? Who will make dinner? These questions come up even during a brief hospitalization.
>
> It's OK to say you don't know the answer to a question. This is often the reality with cancer—we may not know why something happened or what is going to happen next.
>
> You don't have to share everything at once. Several shorter conversations are often better than one long conversation.

Be honest. Don't promise what you may not be able to keep.

Encourage your kids to ask questions and set aside time for that purpose.

Reassure them that cancer is not passed from one person to another. Nothing they did caused your cancer nor can they get cancer from you.

Let them know about your treatment and any expected side effects. If you're going to lose your hair from chemotherapy, let them know in advance so they won't be surprised.

Inform your children's school about your cancer so the teachers can be supportive and be alert for potential changes in behavior.

Sometimes children will ask the difficult question, "Are you going to die?" Breastcancer.org provides an illustration of a good answer: "The doctors have told me that my chances of being cured are very good. I'm going to believe that until I have reason to believe something else. I want you to believe that too. I'll tell you if that changes."

We all want these conversations to go perfectly, but don't be hard on yourself if you get tongue-tied or emotional. It's a hard time for everyone. Kids understand that, too.

Telling the Parents

I've seen many resources that provide advice on how to tell your children that you have cancer.

But what about the other generation—your parents?

Family relationships are sometimes complicated, so I don't presume to know what's best for you and your family, but some guidelines might be helpful.

In general, it's a good idea to talk openly with your parents about your cancer. Keeping secrets consumes energy when you could better use that energy for your own healing. And, if you don't tell your parents, someone else probably will.

But be prepared for your parents having a very emotional response to your cancer diagnosis, even if it's a cancer that's routinely curable. They will hear the word "cancer" and immediately assume the worst. Losing a child is a parent's worst fear.

Telling your parents might even uncover useful information about your family's medical history. A generation ago, there was a much greater stigma attached to cancer, so it wasn't often discussed, even within the family. Maybe they never told you that your grandmother and several aunts had breast cancer. This kind of information is important and should be shared with your physicians.

Problems sometimes arise with parents because they just want to help. This is especially true if they try to influence treatment decisions or otherwise exert control. You may need to gently remind them that you're the decision-maker on all matters relating to your illness.

This is one time in which it's absolutely OK for you to focus on what's best for you. If having your parents with you during cancer treatment is beneficial, then welcome them with open arms. If having them present is stressful, suggest other ways for them to contribute.

Tell them that they can always help by sending good thoughts and positive energy. But do try to keep them in the information loop. Everyone feels better when they're included.

What to Say—and Not Say

Most people find it awkward when first talking with a friend or acquaintance who has just been diagnosed with cancer. Even though nearly everyone is well-intentioned, many say things that hurt or mystify more than they comfort.

Based on my own experiences and my conversations with others with cancer, here are some suggestions:

What not to say

Don't worry. You'll be fine. Everyone's natural instinct is to reassure the newly diagnosed that everything will be OK. While encouraging words are welcome, most people just diagnosed with cancer will be worried. Rather than dismissing those worries, acknowledge them. Honest conversation is likely to follow.

That's too bad about your cancer, but I could be hit by a bus tomorrow. No one in the history of civilization has ever found comfort in these words, but people say it all the time.

Do you smoke? People with lung cancer get asked this routinely. This is blaming, not supporting. People seem to ask this question for their own peace of mind. "You smoked and got lung cancer. I don't smoke, therefore I don't have to worry."

You have to see this doctor or have this treatment or begin this cancer-fighting diet. If people want your advice, they'll ask for it.

Tell me how I can help. This comment often comes from the heart, but it puts the burden on the person with cancer to think of and assign tasks. It's far better just to do things. Bring meals, take care of the kids for an evening, walk the dog, write cards of support, or call and say, "I'm heading to the supermarket. What can I pick up for you? "

What to say

I'm so sorry. This is a good and honest response.

How are you doing with all of this? A simple question like this lets the person with cancer take the lead and opens the door for conversation.

Would you like to grab a cup of coffee and talk?

I'm keeping you in my thoughts and prayers. Positive energy always helps, in whatever form works for you and the person with cancer.

One friend describes two layers of response whenever she tells someone that she has cancer. The first layer is immediate, honest and from the gut. *"Oh no. I'm so sorry."* The second layer is when the person begins saying those things they *think* they should say. *"You'll be fine. You'll be playing tennis in a month."* She wishes that people would stop talking after the "I'm so sorry."

As with other difficult conversations, the specific words are less important than the tangible presence of friends and loved ones. It's OK if the words get a bit tangled—it's the heart that matters.

When a Loved One Has Cancer

A cancer diagnosis changes your life and the lives of the people who love you. It can be especially challenging for your loved ones because they may want to appear strong and optimistic even though they're scared to death on the inside.

In addition to worrying about their loved one's cancer, they may be running the household, struggling with piles of incomprehensible insurance forms, communicating with far-flung family members, and trying to earn enough money to pay the mounting bills. Life doesn't get much more stressful.

I talk with many people who acknowledge this stress, but who also say that helping their loved one through cancer was the best thing they ever did.

What's essential is to understand that the role of the loved one is to support and comfort, not to "fix" the problem. Men tend to have a harder time with this because we somehow expect ourselves to fix whatever is broken. Cancer isn't always fixable.

When people are diagnosed with cancer, they don't want their loved ones to say, "I promise you that you'll be cured." Nobody can guarantee that. Further, that kind of statement cuts off more honest dialogue.

What they want to hear is, "I love you and I'll be here with you for whatever comes."

It's OK to be scared and share that with one another. That's real.

That's one thing about cancer—it's all too real. There's no getting around the fact that it's a bad disease and that there are many unknowns. Sharing that reality will make it more manageable for both of you.

There are things the loved ones can do for their own well-being.

> Carve out some time for yourself, even a few minutes each day. Exercise is especially beneficial because it burns off tension, improves your sleep, and recharges your body.

> Create an outlet where you can talk about you on a regular basis. Therapists, pastors, and long-time friends are good sources of support. Don't try to do everything yourself. Accept offers of help.

There's no way to make caring for a seriously ill loved one easy or painless. It can be exhausting at best and absolutely harrowing at worst. But for many of us, it's the single most courageous and important act of our lives.

Thoughts and Prayer Tree

There's a small tree in the living room of Gary and Mary Ellen Stewart's house in Ithaca. It's covered with cards, letters and drawings.

At first, a visitor isn't quite sure what it is. It looks somewhat like a Christmas tree, but it's the wrong time of year.

A closer look reveals that everything attached to the tree is offering some form of encouragement. "We're thinking of you." "I'm with you." "I love you."

Gary had the idea of creating this "Thoughts and Prayer Tree" to support Mary Ellen who's nearing the end of chemotherapy. Anyone who has been through chemo—or any cancer treatment—can tell you it's a grueling experience that depletes one's spirits and energy.

Friends and family kept asking Gary how they could help Mary Ellen. He suggested that everyone send cards, letters and other expressions of support. These soon began arriving and Gary used twist-ties to attach them to a small, artificial Christmas tree. Gary then took a photo of the tree and sent it out by e-mail which generated many more cards and letters that were then added.

I tend to stack cards in a pile on the coffee table and leave them there for six weeks when I guiltily stick them into the recycling bin. The Thoughts and Prayer Tree, however, lets these cards and letter become living, three-dimensional expressions of support to be read and savored by everyone in the room.

Mary Ellen told me that the cards and letters were personal and deeply felt, unlike Christmas cards which often feel mass produced. She was especially touched by cards from people who were dealing with their own illnesses and challenges, but still took the time to reach out and connect with her.

Another special group of cards, often handmade, were from children who would often stop by the Stewart house to visit the tree. They were always so pleased to see their handiwork displayed.

Gary remarked that it's such a good lesson for children, including their 13-year-old son, Ben, who can see how people can and do support one another through difficult times.

I love the idea of a Thoughts and Prayer Tree. It's both simple and powerful.

It also highlights an important lesson. So often we think of someone or pray for someone who's ill or otherwise in need of our support. But we don't always take the time to actually tell them that we're thinking of them or praying for them. We should.

As I was leaving their home, Mary Ellen gazed up at the tree and said, "I never get tired of looking at it."

During Treatment

Keeping Yourself in Balance

Yesterday afternoon, a woman about to begin chemotherapy came into my office and asked, "What advice do you have to help me get through my treatment?" I've been asked this question in various forms hundreds of times. I now realize that the answer boils down to this: "Keep things in balance."

It's all about being reasonable. I hesitate to make reference to "common sense," because common sense is gained through experience and cancer is new to everyone the first time through.

Here are some examples:

> **Activity level**: I've known some patients to remain flat on their backs throughout months of chemotherapy while others push themselves to compete in athletic events the day after treatment. In general, *moderate* activity is good and either extreme is counterproductive. Too little activity makes fatigue worse, and too much activity drains energy when it's needed for healing. Walking is often more beneficial than either sitting or running.
>
> **Information-seeking**: Some people want to know *everything* about their cancer and its treatment while others want to know as little as possible. Information is almost always helpful, especially when it helps people understand what to expect. You don't want to be surprised when your hair falls out. But too much information can be as harmful as too little information. I've seen people become paralyzed from studying long lists of potential side effects or from getting fifth and sixth medical opinions.

Calling the doctor: Cancer treatment invariably causes side effects. Some side effects are serious and others are more of a nuisance. At one extreme are patients who call the doctor's office ten times a day. At the other extreme are people who never call, even if experiencing fever, pain, or other serious problems. Nurses are great at explaining which side effects are routine and expected, and which ones require attention that day. Take these instructions to heart.

Cancer 24/7: Some patients focus on their cancer 24 hours a day. It's all they talk and think about. Other patients never discuss their cancer and essentially deny that they have it, even in the midst of treatment. One can acknowledge cancer and deal with it, but also take a break from it from time to time. Go out to a movie or dinner and talk about anything *but* cancer for a few hours.

Sense of Control: Cancer is unpredictable and we often lose our sense of control. During treatment, patients are reassured that problems will be addressed if and when they occur. That seems reactive rather than proactive and it makes people uneasy. Sometimes, though, patients (and their families) just need to, well, chill. But it's a mistake to become overly passive and not control what *can* be controlled. Most patients can control how they spend their time and how they take care of themselves. One man put it like this, "I'm letting my doctors work on the cancer. I'm working on making my body healthier."

Every situation and every person is different, so there are no hard and fast rules for all of this. But I think the concepts of balance and moderation during cancer treatment are useful. When people are at one extreme or the other, they tend to experience more problems and more stress. Cancer is never easy, but keeping yourself in balance will make it more manageable.

Non-Traditional Cancer Therapies

People often fall into two camps regarding the usefulness of non-traditional cancer therapies. Some people are irrationally exuberant in their support of these therapies. "This dandelion soup is going to cure my cancer!" Others are completely dismissive. As is usually the case, a balanced perspective is more sensible than either extreme.

These therapies include acupuncture, diet, exercise, massage, yoga, stress management, spiritual pursuits, aromatherapy, and many others. Sometimes they're collectively referred to as alternative medicine or complementary medicine. Increasingly, the term "integrative medicine" is used.

The potential benefits and risks of any type of treatment—conventional or alternative—are especially significant with cancer because the stakes are so high. The choices a person makes can literally mean life or death.

Here's my take on the topic:

When people are diagnosed with cancer, they often feel a loss of control. Nearly anything a person can do to regain some sense of control is understandable. Pursuing non-traditional treatment is an active process and I think that's healthy.

Going through cancer is easier if one is part of a supportive community. I often see such communities emerge naturally from yoga classes, prayer circles, and exercise programs.

Don't force non-traditional modalities on others. The goal is to increase the patient's sense of control, not diminish it.

Michael Lerner's book, *Choices in Healing*, is one of the most thoughtful and balanced books on the topic. He examines alternative approaches to cancer treatment and concludes that there's little evidence that alternative approaches cure cancer, but they may make the patient healthier. A healthier patient is better able to tolerate conventional treatments such as chemotherapy and radiation. And a healthier immune system surely can't hurt.

It's odd that some people think of good nutrition and exercise as alternative approaches to cancer care. They shouldn't be. Eating a well-balanced diet with less meat and more plant-based food is good for nearly everyone. And there's compelling evidence that exercise reduces the likelihood of recurrence for some cancers.

Some alternative approaches (e.g., massage) make a person feel better. As someone who's been through cancer treatment, I can say that anything that makes you feel better is a good thing.

Our organs and diseases don't exist in isolation. Maybe yoga won't directly affect your cancer, but it may affect your emotional well-being which, in turn, can affect your cardiovascular system.

Don't begin radical lifestyle changes when beginning cancer treatment. There will be times when you'll need to sit on the couch and eat ice cream. That's OK. You need that rest and those calories.

Tell your doctors about your alternative approaches, even something that seems as benign as taking vitamins. This is especially true during chemotherapy. Antioxidants are usually good for people because they help keep cells alive, but chemotherapy is trying to kill cancer cells. The antioxidants can prevent the chemo from working. Other vitamins can affect how the body heals from surgery.

In sum, when thinking about non-traditional cancer modalities, the most important question isn't, "Will this treatment cure my cancer?" Rather, the question to ask, "Will this treatment contribute to my health and well-being?"

Doctor-Patient Interactions

I spend much of my time helping seriously ill patients navigate the health care system. As a result, I'm constantly talking with patients about their interactions with doctors and other health professionals.

Although each encounter is unique, I'm increasingly aware of some universal truths that contribute to good patient-doctor encounters. Not surprisingly, good encounters require a shared spirit of respect and communication.

I've found most providers in our area to be committed to patient care and quality service. But all of us can benefit from gentle reminders from time to time.

Suggestions for doctors and other health professionals

Introduce yourself to new patients. This should be obvious, but it doesn't always happen.

Listen for a while without interrupting. Get the big picture before filling in the details. This is often more of a problem in offices that use electronic medical records. Focus on the patient and not on the computer screen, especially during the first few minutes of the visit.

Be kind.

Remind yourself that patients newly diagnosed with a serious illness are scared. If you deal with sick people every day, it becomes routine. It's not routine for the new patient.

> Make a special effort to establish communication and a sense of partnership during the initial visit. Subsequent visits will benefit.
>
> Respect that patients may have beliefs—about health care, about life priorities, about whatever—that differ from your own. A decision that's wrong for you may not be wrong for them.
>
> Recognize that medical care is costly for most people, even those with good insurance. The best medicine won't help if the patient can't afford to fill the prescription.
>
> Make good communication between patients and the entire office staff an ongoing priority. Few offices do this really well and every office could do it better.

Suggestions for patients

> Recognize that you are not your doctor's only patient.
>
> Respect your doctor's time. If you have multiple questions, ask the most important questions first.
>
> Don't think of your doctor as the enemy. If you don't like your doctor, get a new one. Everyone will be happier.
>
> Be honest and open about your medical history and your present concerns. Don't make your doctor guess.
>
> Recognize that good health is largely your responsibility. Eat sensibly. Exercise. Don't smoke.
>
> Recognize that medicine is not a perfect science. A bad outcome does not mean bad care.

Be reasonable. And be polite.

Good health care *is* a partnership. It's all about communication and respect. And it flows in both directions.

A Better Phrase than Staying Strong

If your loved one has cancer, you may sense an obligation to be strong. The phrase "Be strong" is branded into our brains, but I wish we had a better phrase to capture the role of the people closest to those with cancer.

Being strong makes me think of Clint Eastwood characters. Never flinching, always moving forward, threatening to beat cancer to a pulp. I, for one, would not be comforted by having Dirty Harry in my chemotherapy room.

Strong sometimes gets confused with stoic. A man in treatment once told me, "My wife tries to be strong and not cry in front of me, but we both know it's an act. We've been married for 45 years and she always cries. It's just who she is. I wish she would cry with me now."

When everyone else goes home, you need to have someone stay behind and share your reality. With cancer, the reality is sometimes good, sometimes bad, and often uncertain.

I think a better phrase than "being strong" is "being connected." That's what a person with cancer most needs—the sense that a loved one will be there and be connected for whatever comes.

One critical role for the loved one is to focus on the patient's quality of life—is treatment affecting the patient's ability to sleep? To eat? Are they experiencing pain? Sometimes doctors—and even patients—need to be reminded about the seemingly small things that can make a huge difference in how the person feels. I recently heard one person describe his spouse as his "quality of life advocate."

He went on to say that everyone needs a quality of life advocate during cancer treatment. I couldn't agree more.

Advocating for a Loved One

I've often written that it is helpful for a person with cancer to have an advocate present during doctor's appointments and hospital stays. I'd like to devote this column to the nuts and bolts of what this really means. What I describe is based on seeing hundreds of loved ones serving as advocates. Nearly all are well-intentioned, but not all are effective or even helpful.

The most important role for the advocate is to understand and be supportive of the patient and the patient's wishes.

Above all, a good advocate needs to be a good listener. Listen to the patient. And listen to the health professionals.

Most problems occur when loved ones confuse their own wishes and agenda with those of the patient. This isn't done maliciously. More often, it's based on assumptions of what's best for the patient without actually *asking* the patient.

It's entirely normal for loved ones to have their own agendas. But understand that the patient's agenda and loved ones' agendas aren't necessarily one and the same.

It can be helpful for patients and their loved ones to separately write down their wishes and priorities. Afterwards, compare the lists to see where they overlap and where they differ. This provides clarity and also a springboard for discussion.

Ultimately, though, advocates need to realize that it is the patient and the patient's wishes that take precedence.

Here are a few additional suggestions for advocates:

The Elephant in the Room

Talk with the patient before appointments to write down questions the patient wants to ask.

Let the patient speak for him or herself.

Take notes.

Let the health care team do its work.

Report changes in the patient's status to the health professionals, especially ones that aren't obvious. For example, "Sarah seems to have much less energy than she did last month."

Understand the reality of the situation and maintain reasonable expectations.

Think of yourself as part of the care team. Ask both the patient and the professionals how you can be helpful.

Be a bridge-builder. Connect with providers, other patients and family members.

Think of ways to help with non-medical issues, e.g., household chores, that free up the patient's time and energy.

Some people don't think of themselves as advocates because they aren't loud and pushy. In fact, the best advocates are quiet forces who support mostly by their steadfast presence. I heard one patient refer to his advocate as his "designated listener." What a perfect description. We should all have designated listeners.

Groundhog Friends

I'm often asked how to be a friend to someone with cancer.

I generally answer this question by encouraging them to be good listeners and to be present for their friend in every sense of the word.

This being the first week in February, I describe it as being a "groundhog friend."

Remember the movie *Groundhog Day* with Bill Murray? The same day kept reappearing. That isn't a good trait for one's day, but it's a terrific trait in a friend of someone with cancer.

When you're first diagnosed, many people call, send notes, and help in a variety of ways. That's great and those kindnesses are appreciated.

But cancer is more a marathon than a sprint. The challenging time is when the initial outpouring of support slows and you still have four months of chemotherapy looming ahead.

A groundhog friend checks on you throughout the course of your treatment.

A groundhog friend keeps sending notes of support.

A groundhog friend keeps popping up to do things that make your life easier.

A groundhog friend isn't offended by your crankiness on those inevitable bad days.

A groundhog friend doesn't change the subject when you have bad news to share.

A groundhog friend keeps filling your freezer with food.

A groundhog friend brings in other friends when you're in the mood and keeps them away when you aren't.

Above all, a groundhog friend keeps reappearing, day after day.

Helping from a Distance

I once received a letter from a man serving time in prison asking how he could help his mother who was ill with cancer.

As I wrote back to offer suggestions, I recall thinking that this was an extreme example of long-distance caregiving. He literally couldn't visit his mother and his ability to communicate with her was limited.

There are countless other situations in which someone wants to help a loved one with cancer, but geography makes it impossible to pop over with a bowl of soup and a hug.

But there *are* ways to help and support, even if you can't be there in person:

- Send notes of support. Let them know that you're sending positive thoughts.

- Realize that people with cancer often receive lots of cards when they are first diagnosed. The cards that they receive weeks and months later—when they're tired of cancer and its treatment—are especially treasured.

- Don't be discouraged if you don't receive a response. People in the middle of treatment often need to conserve their energy. I've known people to respond seemingly out of the blue years later to say how much those cards meant.

- Educate yourself about their cancer. Lung cancer is very different than breast cancer. Acquiring a basic knowledge will help you understand what they're going through and facilitate communication.

Call, even if it feels awkward at first. It's OK to say simply, "I'm sorry you have cancer." People don't usually remember what you said, but they'll remember that you called. And don't worry about waking someone up or disturbing them. They have an answering machine.

Small gifts, unrelated to illness, are always welcome.

Reach out to the primary caregiver. They may need an outlet. Or simply a recognition of their difficult role.

I've had friends take part in cancer walks and raise money in my honor. I love when that happens.

If writing or calling is difficult, you can always send good and positive thoughts. As one friend with cancer told me, "Prayers, good vibes, thinking of me—I'll take it in any form."

More than anything, the person with cancer will appreciate the sense of staying connected with you and staying connected with his or her "normal" life. Cancer tends to throw everything into upheaval. Distant friends and family can help people with cancer maintain their sense of who they were before cancer and, hopefully, the life to which they will return when treatment ends.

Helping Those We Don't Like

In my columns, I often suggest practical ways to help people with cancer. Giving support to nice people is relatively easy. You want to bring them soup and give them a hug.

But contrary to what you see in the movies, not everyone with cancer is angelic. Some of us are cranky. Others are downright unpleasant.

Whether one likes them or not, unpleasant people need support, too.

In my experience, unpleasant people with cancer were unpleasant people before they had cancer. And nothing about cancer is going to make them any happier.

The first unpleasant person who comes to your mind might be a member of your family. Perhaps it's a parent or a sibling. Or it could be a neighbor, member of your faith community, or coworker.

If this unpleasant person gets cancer, you may feel some obligation to help. This sense of obligation might be heightened if the person is socially isolated which, not surprisingly, tends to happen to unpleasant people.

So, what to do?

My suggestion is to reach out to them by calling, visiting, and offering to take them to appointments. But don't expect them to smile, be gracious, or appreciate your assistance.

We're taught by Hollywood that cranky people have hearts of gold and twinkles in their eyes. I've known several people like that, but I've also known people who seem to have hearts of stone, and the word "twinkle" will never, ever be used to describe them.

Henri Nouwen provided a perfect description of support and caring:

> When we honestly ask ourselves which persons in our lives mean the most to us, we often find that it is those who, instead of giving advice, solutions, or cures, have chosen rather to share our pain and touch our wounds with a warm and tender hand. The friend who can be silent with us in a moment of despair or confusion, who can stay with us in an hour of grief and bereavement, who can tolerate not knowing, not curing, not healing and face with us the reality of our powerlessness, that is a friend who cares.

Providing that kind of support even to our loved ones is difficult. Providing that kind of support to someone who's unpleasant is next to impossible.

But that doesn't mean that we can't help in one way or another, even if it's a small gesture and we have to force a smile.

A friend of mine, referring to her sister, put it to me this way, "I don't like her, but I'm here for her."

There's a lot of wisdom and love in that statement. Sometimes we help simply because it's the right thing to do.

Practical Ways to Help

One of my recent columns cautioned against giving unsolicited advice to friends who have cancer.

A reader called and said, "OK, I won't give unsolicited advice. But what *can* I do to help my neighbor who just found out she has cancer?"

It's a great question. I began my answer with a preface: don't expect to make things all better. You can't. But you can always do something to make life better for your friend on any given day:

Drive her to doctor appointments or treatments.

Drop off a meal that can be easily frozen for future use.

If she wants to talk about cancer, let her do so without interruption.

If she does not want to talk about cancer, take her to a movie.

Offer to organize other friends who also want to help by cooking or driving.

If many calls are expected, offer to answer the phone and relay information.

If she's a neighbor, just go ahead and cut her grass, weed her garden, or fill her birdfeeders.

Offer to do research. It can be as straightforward as calling around to see which store in the area has the best price for an item that she'll need.

Take walks with her.

Buy her a 6-month subscription to Netflix.

Offer to watch her kids for an evening or weekend.

Write her notes of encouragement and support, especially later in her treatment when others write less often.

Send photos and other reminders of happy times together.

Send small gifts—a favorite book or CD.

Don't take offense if your friend doesn't call you back right away. Being treated for cancer is a full-time job that uses up a lot of energy. Take the initiative for staying in touch. Understand that your friend's needs and wishes will change during treatment and recovery. If she doesn't want to go out for lunch now, ask again next month. And the month after.

Chemobrain

Some people report memory loss, slower mental processing speed, and other cognitive changes after chemotherapy. Anyone who has been in a cancer support group has heard these symptoms described as *chemobrain* or *chemofog*, but only recently have researchers and clinicians given it much attention. It turns out to be a complicated issue because so many factors may be involved.

Nearly every cancer patient experiences fatigue and stress, and a significant number report some degree of depression, all of which can affect a person's memory and ability to think clearly. And cancer is most common in individuals over the age of 65, a time when cognitive changes might appear independently of cancer or its treatment. Measuring cognitive changes specifically caused by chemotherapy is difficult.

Most existing studies relating to chemobrain are small, tend to focus only on individuals being treated for breast cancer, and have used inconsistent measures. As a result, we don't have much solid data that can be generalized. The International Cognition and Cancer Task Force has been formed to tackle this issue. One of its highest prioritize is to standardize measures so that studies can be compared and synthesized.

I had chemotherapy more than a decade ago and I experienced what I consider to be chemobrain. It didn't affect my day-to-day functioning, but it did seem to hamper my ability to kick my brain into its highest gear. For a college professor—which I was at the time—losing high gear can be a serious problem. Fortunately, the symptoms disappeared in a few months as they do for most people. In some cases, though, chemobrain seems to linger on for years.

A recent article in the *Journal of the National Cancer Institute* calls for the adoption of a term more encompassing than chemobrain. Cognitive changes in cancer patients can be caused by treatments other than chemotherapy (e.g., hormonal therapy, immunotherapy, and radiation therapy) or by the cancer itself.

So what does this all mean for someone just now diagnosed with cancer? Here's my take:

Realize that most people undergoing chemotherapy do not experience cognitive problems. The Mayo Clinic website estimates that twenty to thirty percent of people undergoing chemotherapy will experience problems.

If your brain seems fuzzy when you're getting cancer treatment, report these symptoms to your doctor. Some problems can be corrected by changing medications or some other relatively easy fix.

If you feel depressed, share that with your doctor. A Lance Armstrong Foundation survey of cancer survivors found that seventy percent of them experienced depression at some point in time. Depression is treatable.

Exercise during treatment is often helpful. Aerobic activity can clear your mind and make you feel more alert.

In sum, there is a growing recognition that cognitive changes sometime occur as a result of cancer and its treatment, but we don't know exactly why it happens or who is at greatest risk. In general, these changes are transient and manageable, but we're just beginning to understand the scope of the problem and what to do about it.

More than Tired

When people think about the side effects of cancer treatment, they usually think about hair loss (which is common with some types of chemotherapy), and nausea (which is not nearly as common as it used to be). In my mind, though, fatigue is the side effect of cancer treatment that's both most universal and least appreciated.

Fatigue is different than simply being tired. People often describe it as a complete loss of energy. I hear the phrases, "dead tired" or "bone tired" all of the time. Washing the dishes can seem like climbing Mount Everest. And people often wake up in the morning feeling just as depleted. Fatigue is more than a nuisance, it can completely disrupt one's life.

Some causes of cancer-related fatigue are organic and respond well to treatment. Anemia, for example, is sometimes caused by chemotherapy. If people don't have enough red blood cells, they won't feel very peppy. Anemia can be treated.

Sometimes fatigue is caused by simply not eating enough. Treatment (and cancer itself) can affect a person's appetite or ability to swallow. Nutritionists can help identify foods and supplements that are both palatable and provide enough calories. Medication can be used to stimulate a person's appetite if it continues to be a problem.

Sleep is often disrupted during cancer treatment. A person's life rhythms get out of whack—they go to bed at odd hours, nap during the day, and worry at regular intervals. The medications themselves can affect sleep cycles. A good night's sleep restores both a person's body and emotions. If sleep is a problem, talk with your doctor about medication and/or other solutions.

Depression is common for many people with cancer and depression can independently affect sleep, appetite, and energy. Sometimes it's hard to sort out what's causing what. Is depression causing the fatigue, or is it cancer treatment? When a person is in middle of treatment and suffering significant side effects, if often makes sense to see what works, even if the cause isn't completely understood. Addressing the depression often helps.

For many, the cause of fatigue is the lack of activity. It's easy to become out of shape after months of surgery, chemo, and radiation. It's a vicious cycle in that fatigue can cause one to stay on the couch which, in turn, causes more fatigue. Gentle exercise, such as walking, is almost always helpful.

Even when the fatigued can't be "fixed," it can be managed. One nurse tells her patients that it's like beginning each day with $100 in their energy bank. Once it's gone for the day, it's gone, so they need to prioritize their activities. At the top of the list are things that have to get done as well as those things that provide the greatest pleasure. Other activities can wait or friends can be called in to help with the dishes or shop for groceries. Friends who want to help are often delighted to have concrete tasks assigned.

Cancer-related fatigue is just beginning to receive the attention it deserves. Just as pain assessment has become a standardized and regular component of medical care, fatigue assessment is entering the realm of routine cancer care. One survey of cancer patients found that most experienced fatigue, but few discussed it with their physicians. I hope this soon changes. Just like pain, fatigue can be overwhelming and debilitating. It can and should be addressed as a matter of course.

Understanding Friends with Cancer

I recently had a conversation with someone whose good friend was diagnosed with cancer. She hoped that the cancer wouldn't change their friendship, but it did. The change, though, was temporary. As she told me, "My friend had to go through a process to come to terms with her cancer— I just didn't understand that at first."

When people are diagnosed with a life-threatening illness, they aren't sure what they should think, and they're even less sure what they should say to family and friends. It's a period of emotional churning more than of clear insight. Most people need time to sort things out in their own minds before discussing it with anyone outside of their immediate families.

But friends often want to know some of the specifics of the patient's condition and the proposed treatment. Imagine having a long-time friend that you've shared *everything* with. All of sudden, she has cancer and she's not talking. It's easy to feel left out.

As this person told me, "I wondered if she was telling other people about her cancer, but not me. I felt out of the loop."

Several weeks later, though, this person realized that, "This has to be about her, not about me." She was feeling left out because she was focusing on her own needs and not on the needs of the person with cancer. Once this realization hit, she was able to relax and let her friend's internal process take its natural course.

She decided to be a silent friend, to listen, to be available, to be supportive, but not to pry. She left flowers on her doorstop, sent cards and remained a steady presence. In turn, her friend called on her more and more because she knew that she wouldn't get questions that she didn't want to answer.

This is how Rachel Naomi Remen described this gift of listening, "The most basic and powerful way to connect to another person is to listen. Just listen. Perhaps the most important thing we ever give each other is our attention . . . . A loving silence often has far more power to heal and to connect than the most well-intentioned words."

And gentle silence often leads to honest conversations when the time is right. When her friend with cancer was ready to talk, the floodgates opened wide.

There was so much that her friend had to say, but it just wasn't time until that particular moment.

Cancer can and does change friendships, but the best friendships are resilient and will re-emerge after a period of adjustment. To be a true friend is to respect the privacy, process, and timetable of the person with cancer. When in doubt, just listen with an open heart.

Visiting Those in the Hospital

People with cancer are sometimes hospitalized and their friends often want to visit to offer support and encouragement. Understanding some general guidelines will help make the visit a positive experience for everyone:

- Keep the visits brief. People in the hospital are generally quite ill and have limited energy. If you stay long, it puts a burden on them to keep you entertained. Visits of ten to fifteen minutes are often best.

- Be sure that the patient wants visitors. Call ahead to see if visiting is a good idea and, if so, what time of day is preferred.

- If a visit isn't possible, send a card. And bring a card with you if you do visit. Patients often put those cards on the wall and feel comforted by them.

- Don't visit if you're sick. The last thing a hospitalized patient needs is your germs.

- Wash your hands before entering the room, even if you're healthy. There are sinks and alcohol-based hand cleansers throughout the hospital. Use them.

- Don't wear strong fragrances. Some ill patients are acutely sensitive to scents. And please don't smoke before visiting—the smell lingers on your clothes.

- If doctors or other health professionals enter the room, excuse yourself and go into the hallway unless the patient specifically asks that you stay.

The Elephant in the Room

If family members are present, realize that the patient needs private time with them. Give your regards, but don't linger in the room.

Don't sit on the patient's bed unless you are asked to do so. Patients are often physically uncomfortable and they don't want to be jostled or cramped.

Don't hug the patient unless it's clear that they want that hug. If you've just had surgery, a hug is painful.

Don't whine about things in your life. No one wants to hear, "I'm sorry that you have lung cancer, Joe, but I just got a parking ticket and I'm really steamed."

Don't pry into the patient's health. If they want to share with you, they'll share with you. It's fine to ask how they're feeling, but leave it at that.

Don't be afraid of silence. Sometimes it's the best support you can provide.

As is so often the case, what's in your heart is more important than the words you say. When people are seriously ill, they sense kindness and support around them. Your visits, cards, prayers, and positive thoughts do make a difference.

Single with Cancer

For a day or two following chemotherapy, most people camp out on the couch and do nothing more strenuous than watch TV or flip through magazines.

Loved ones bring glasses of water, cups of tea, and small snacks to lift the patient's spirits and provide nourishment.

If you're single, going through cancer treatment can be especially challenging. If you don't get off the couch to fetch your own water, you may go thirsty.

You also worry about who's going to drive you to doctor appointments, relay information to relatives and friends, do the grocery shopping, and walk the dog.

There are financial issues: if you can't work, you don't get paid. Even short-term absences from work can be difficult. Your income may go down just as your expenses go up. There's no cushion of a second income or a spouse's health insurance.

And who's going to be with you in those dark moments when everyone else goes home? It's scary when it's quiet and your mind inevitably wonders to those "what if" questions.

Perhaps you're in a new romantic relationship or simply looking forward to future relationships. Cancer tends to complicate all of this. Potential changes in body image, fertility, and even life expectancy can be very big elephants in the room.

But all is not gloom. A recurring theme in my columns is that people are remarkably resilient, and that is certainly true for most single people with cancer.

Some single people I know actually prefer going through cancer treatment alone. They like having the freedom to focus strictly on their own needs and "not putting on a happy face for others."

And, of course, not every marriage or partnership is a good one. Having an unsupportive partner during cancer treatment might well be worse than having no partner at all.

Although cancer can complicate new relationships, it can be a positive force as well. I've seen several relationships (both romantic and otherwise) take root during and after cancer treatment. When you have cancer, you tend to worry less about the small stuff and appreciate the good that's around you.

Often the good around you comes in the form of dear friends who step up and support you in your journey.

But when there's no one to help fetch that glass of water, you do it yourself. And you continue to move forward.

Cancer as a Marathon

Chris LaVallee will soon run a 7-day, 155-mile race in the Australian wilderness to raise funds for the Cancer Resource Center of the Finger Lakes.

I recently heard him describe the race and his training and then answer questions from an audience of supporters. One asked, "How do you keep going mentally when your body is exhausted?"

As Chris began to answer, I realized that distance running is a perfect metaphor for cancer treatment.

Anyone who has had cancer can tell you that it's a marathon, not a sprint.

At the starting line, everyone is pumped up because of the cheering crowd and the uncertainty of what lies ahead.

The challenge is when the starting line is far behind and the finish line isn't yet in sight. Physical and mental fatigue can be overwhelming.

Distance runners expect this fatigue and train for it. Their coaches prepare them to "run through it."

People with cancer rarely have the opportunity to train before beginning treatment. And they're likely to be more concerned about losing their hair, throwing up, and dying than about fatigue.

But they're surprised to find that fatigue is often the most disruptive side effect of treatment. There's the physical fatigue that sometimes makes getting out of bed a challenge.

And then there's the mental fatigue. If the first four cycles of chemotherapy knocked you on your butt, you know the fifth cycle won't be any easier.

Just as runners appreciate those who cheer them on far into the race, people with cancer especially appreciate their supporters who cheer them on far into treatment. There's always a crowd at the starting line and the finish line. We most remember the solitary cheerleader who gives us a lift when we most need it.

Many people with early cancer receive chemotherapy and/or radiation for a set period of time to reduce the risk of a recurrence. There's a clear finish line.

But people with more advanced cancers often receive chemotherapy on an ongoing basis to keep their cancers under control. This is like being a distance runner in a long race without a clear finish line. They just keep running. I really admire their, well, athleticism.

Let's all give a cheer to Chris as heads off to run that 155-mile race in Australia. And let's cheer as well for our family members, friends, and neighbors as they face the challenges of cancer with strength and perseverance.

Holiday Gifts

I have been thinking about gift suggestions for people who are being treated for cancer and for those who have recently completed treatment.

As a starting point, my recommendation is to give gifts of life rather than gifts of cancer. No matter how well-intentioned the gift, I become cranky if I find my stocking stuffed with pink ribbons or books with titles like, "Cancer is a Special Blessing" or "I Beat Cancer with an Eggplant and Zucchini Diet."

Give people an opportunity to think about something other than cancer.

In addition to everything else, cancer is expensive and disposable money is often tight. Give little luxuries. A gift certificate to a favorite restaurant or to a local theater can be a real treat. Join together with friends and give a person a day of pampering at a local spa. If they have an iPod, give a gift certificate so they can download their favorite tunes.

Sometimes, basic necessities are needed most of all. Something as simple as a gas card to help pay for trips back and forth for treatment can give a family a little breathing space.

For the person who's completed treatment, consider something with a future orientation. The time immediately following treatment is often unexpectedly difficult, so help them look ahead. Perhaps tickets to a play that's coming to town in a few months or an upcoming sporting event.

The Elephant in the Room

Many people who have had a life-threatening illness recommit to making their lives as meaningful as possible. Consider making a donation to their favorite charity in their honor.

You can also give of yourself in a very tangible way. You can register with the National Marrow Donor Program (1-800-627-7692) to help people with leukemia, lymphoma, and other diseases that can be treated by a bone marrow transplant.

Finally, make it a point to send cards and call people who have been affected by cancer and tell them that they are in your thoughts, not only during the holiday season, but throughout the year.

Holiday Gifts for those with Serious Illness

I once wrote a column on buying holiday gifts for people with cancer. I discouraged gifts that focused on illness. No one I know wants a stocking stuffer titled, "Prunes and Persimmons: Fighting Your Cancer with Foods that Begin with P."

I recommended gifts with a future orientation—tickets for upcoming concerts or perhaps a trip to somewhere pleasant. Thinking about life *after* cancer often brings a smile.

But what if your loved one has advanced cancer and this holiday season may be their last? Gifts with a future orientation might be well-intentioned, but they ignore the elephant in the room.

If your mother is nearing the end of her life, why not celebrate that life?

A photo album or scrapbook that captures your mother's life will have more meaning for her than a new pair of slippers. Ask her friends and other family members to contribute photos and mementoes. They'll be delighted.

And I think it's a wonderful tribute to make donations in a person's honor *before* they die. Suggest donations to your mom's favorite charity, perhaps creating a special fund in her honor.

Some people say that gifts that celebrate a person's life are wrong because they imply the person is dying.

The Elephant in the Room

Hello? If your mom is dying, she knows that she's dying. Giving her a family scrapbook isn't going to push her over the edge.

Holidays bring families together and most of us make special efforts to join loved ones if a family member is seriously ill. Sharing stories is not an admission of impending death—it's a celebration of life and a recognition that a person's life continues to have meaning.

There's no question that holidays take on an added poignancy when a loved one is nearing the end of life. Expect some tears. But expect laughter as well. It's all about life.

When a Partner is in Denial

I recently spoke with a woman who was stressed because her husband has cancer and he seemed to be in denial over the seriousness of his situation.

What was especially upsetting to her was that he didn't want to address any end of life issues like drafting a will.

I've been mulling this over ever since. What happens when a couple faces cancer and they aren't on the same page?

It's sometimes a matter of perspective. Is the glass half-full or half-empty? With a particular cancer, the chance of surviving might be eighty percent. On the other hand, the chance of dying is twenty percent. Different people focus on different numbers.

It can also be a function of timing. Absorbing a diagnosis of cancer doesn't happen overnight and people have to do it at their own pace. Your partner won't necessarily process the news and their accompanying emotions on your timetable.

And realize that a partner's seeming denial might be a useful coping strategy in the short term. It's how they can get through the next few weeks without falling apart.

Here are a few recommendations:

> It is almost always helpful for a couple to attend medical appointments together so they can hear the same news at the same time. It's hard to be in emotionally if you aren't working from the same set of facts.
>
> Be patient with your partner. Listen without judgment.

At the same time, recognize and address your own needs. Joining a support group can provide an emotional outlet and a chance to connect with others in similar situations.

Too much about cancer is uncertain and uncontrollable, so control what you can control. Everyone should have a will and a health care proxy. Take care of them so there are fewer things to worry about. If your spouse balks, say that it's important for your peace of mind and then take the initiative in making the arrangements.

Sometimes the person in denial is the individual with cancer. Just as often, it's the partner of the person with cancer who's the one in denial. Either way, the principles of being patient and supportive of your partner while addressing your own needs works equally well in either situation.

After Treatment

The After-Treatment Blahs

For many people the months following cancer treatment are more difficult than the treatment itself.

During treatment, your "job" is to be in treatment. You're busy with appointments and you see the same doctors and nurses almost every week. At the same time, friends bring you meals, family members take on extra duties, and you're left to focus on getting better.

Then you have your last radiation therapy treatment or chemotherapy session. You get hugs and congratulatory handshakes. There's an expectation that everything in your life will suddenly revert back to normal.

Let me pop that bubble: everything doesn't return to normal right away. You might even wonder, "Is my new normal the same as my old normal?" Your body is tired. Your brain is muddled. You're worried that the cancer will come back. And you miss the safe cocoon of your chemo nurses and radiation therapists.

What makes it especially hard is that the people around you sometimes expect you to bounce back almost immediately. While they were happy to help you during treatment, they now see you as recovered and expect you to carry your old load. "C'mon, Bob. You finished chemo on Friday. We need you at linebacker against the Giants on Sunday." (Maybe I'm fantasizing just a little, but, hey, it's my column.)

The post-treatment blahs are so common that I try to prepare people for them in advance. This is what I suggest:

> Expect a post-treatment slump. Rather than being a time of celebration, the last treatment is sometimes the

beginning of a funk. If you expect that funk, it won't be so difficult.

Realize that recovery is not a straight line. You'll feel better one day but worse the next. That's normal.

Expect recovery to take several months. Some people say that the recovery phase takes as long as the treatment phase. It took me a full year following chemotherapy to really feel like myself again.

Expect to be acutely aware of every ache and pain and immediately think the worst. Every headache is an ominous sign of a brain tumor instead of just a normal headache. Every cough is a lung metastasis instead of a normal cold. These worries become even more pronounced before doctor visits and tests. You scan your body for the slightest indication of anything bad. Everyone goes through this.

Realize that cancer will continue to be front and center in your life for several more months. It's what you think about in the morning, at night, and throughout the day. But this fades with time. The second year after treatment is much easier than the first year after treatment.

Expect your family and friends to have less time to sit with you and listen to your concerns about living with cancer. They're eager to get back to normal as quickly as possible. There's a good chance that you still want to process what you've been through. Joining a support group or speaking with a therapist can be especially helpful during this transition phase.

Most of all, be patient with those around you and especially with yourself.

When Loved Ones Complete Treatment

Most people realize that their loved ones with cancer need special attention when they are beginning treatment.

Fewer people realize that their loved ones also need special attention when they are *finishing* cancer treatment.

Family members generally look forward to the end of treatment because it means that life may get back to normal. They've probably put their own lives on hold for months, and they're eager for a vacation from the whole cancer experience.

People with cancer often have mixed feelings as treatment ends. While they're happy to be rid of the unpleasant side effects of chemotherapy and radiation, they wonder what the future holds. Have they been cured, or will the cancer return?

These fears fade with time, but the months immediately following treatment are especially difficult. Patients miss the security provided by their chemo nurses and radiation therapists. These professionals provide a ready outlet for their questions and fears.

When treatment is over, many patients think about cancer nearly all of the time. They stew over things and they want to talk. The people most likely to be within earshot are loved ones who may be less than enthused about talking about cancer, cancer, and more cancer.

So, how can loved ones help while maintaining their own sanity?

I recommend that they encourage the patient to talk about their feelings, but mostly with someone *other* than a loved one. This is a perfect time for to join a support group. I joined a group when I found myself in a post-treatment funk and that group provided just the outlet I needed.

In addition to face-to-face groups, there are on-line discussion groups for nearly every type of cancer and situation. Some people, of course, just don't like groups, and I encourage them to connect on an individual basis with a therapist, pastor, or other professional who can offer emotional support. This can provide some much-needed breathing space for everyone. In most cases, therapy is not needed on a long-term basis—just during that period of transition immediately following treatment.

Loved ones can also help by gently shifting the focus from illness to wellness. I always caution against making major lifestyle changes *during* cancer treatment, but lifestyle changes *after* treatment often help physically and provide one with a sense of control. And nearly everyone can benefit from a better diet, moderate exercise, and other healthy behaviors.

My purpose in writing this column is not to suggest that loved ones don't do enough. They do plenty. I see them daily in radiation medicine and in the chemo suites, providing support and practical assistance. They make a difficult experience somehow manageable.

But getting back to normal following cancer treatment is a slow process, and reaching for help from outside the family is often in everyone's best interests.

Survivor's Guilt

People going through cancer treatment at the same time often form their own peer group. They see each other in chemo, in radiation, and in various support groups. The fortunate ones do well, but they often feel guilty when others in their cohort succumb to the disease.

Survivor's guilt is a well-known phenomenon, but it's usually thought of in the context of war, disasters, and other catastrophic events. Why does one person live when others perish?

With cancer, it's a slower, more subtle process. There's a gradual realization that many of the people who once gathered together for a support group are no longer living.

Sometimes it's expected. Some cancers clearly have poorer prognoses than others. But sometimes it seems completely arbitrary, especially when a person's "cancer buddies" are those with the same cancer.

I'm not a fan of using military metaphors when writing about cancer, but it may be apt in relation to survivor's guilt. It's difficult to be a survivor if your buddies didn't make it. Survivors often feel more weariness than celebration.

I don't mean to suggest that survivor's guilt is ever-present in the minds of those of us with cancer. It's not. It just flits in and out of our consciousness, especially when another death occurs.

Sometimes it helps just to recognize this guilt and give it a name.

I've found that it's also beneficial to memorialize those who have died. They would be pleased that life continues. Memorials can take the form of donations, participating in cancer walks, volunteering, or simply planting flowers in their honor.

I've often written that cancer brings a profound sense of community. It's really the best thing that came out of my cancer. But by bringing connection, community also brings loss. It's inevitable and often painful.

But that sense of community is so good and so strong. Harold Kushner captured its essence when he wrote, "What cannot be achieved in one lifetime will happen when one lifetime is joined to another."

Post-Cancer Relationships

It's often a challenge to begin a new relationship after you've had cancer. I've written about this in the past as have many others. But these writings almost always focus on the person *with* cancer.

What about the other partner in a new relationship—the one without cancer?

One woman put it this way, "I feel like cancer is a member of his family. I want to understand and help, but he never wants to talk about it."

This reminds me of those old movies in which the newcomer to the household realizes there's a mysterious person living in the attic. This person is never mentioned even though his footsteps are heard from time to time. The newcomer is concerned and curious, but it's clear that questions aren't welcomed.

That's not a good situation in the movies or in real life.

I encourage the partner with cancer to be as open as possible. Some people want to compartmentalize their cancer experience and not think about it again. That doesn't work well if there's a new partner. Like it or not, cancer is part of your life, so share it.

And I encourage the partner without cancer to ask questions. If your partner doesn't want to answer those questions just then, try to schedule a time to sit down and talk it through.

Talking about cancer is scary, but not talking about cancer is even scarier.

New relationships after cancer can be challenging even with good communication.

When a person goes through cancer with a partner, it's generally a shared experience. Together, they learn the language of cancer and mutually understand what's been done and what the future holds. If the relationship develops some time after the cancer diagnosis, the partner without cancer needs to catch up.

For some new couples, the cancer is mostly a distant memory that has little impact. Perhaps a scar and an annual check-up are the only reminders.

For other couples, cancer is a day-to-day presence. Some cancers require ongoing treatment. Even cancers that are presumably cured can have significant aftereffects: changes in body image, colostomies, sexual difficulties, infertility, fatigue. These are real challenges to a new relationship.

I love meeting couples who fall in love in spite of these challenges. If you can work together through cancer, you can work together through anything.

And having had cancer is not all bad. People who have been through serious illness don't take much for granted. Life doesn't have to be perfect to be good.

Donating Blood and Organs

I once wrote a column about fumbling for words when the Red Cross called and asked if I would donate blood. I had just been diagnosed with cancer and found it hard to say, "I have cancer."

After the column appeared, a reader stopped me and asked, "Well, *can* you give blood after having cancer?"

Good question. I promised her that I would find out.

In a similar vein (so to speak), I'm always stumped when asked if I'm an organ donor.

If I check the box, "Yes, I am an organ donor," I worry that whoever gets my kidney will get my breast cancer too.

If I check "No, I am not an organ donor," I feel like I have to justify it by writing, "I'd like to donate, but I've had cancer and they probably wouldn't want my organs anyway." (It's hard to fit all of that on the back of my driver's license.) It turns out that most people who've had cancer can donate both blood and organs.

According to the American Red Cross, a person can give blood if he or she is cancer-free and at least one year has elapsed since the completion of treatment. The waiting time was recently reduced from five years to one year.

Taking tamoxifen (commonly prescribed to prevent a recurrence of breast cancer) and many other drugs do not disqualify a person from giving blood.

The only cancers that prevent a person from donating blood on a permanent basis are leukemia and lymphoma.

An interesting article appeared in the medical journal *Lancet* in May 2007. The researchers identified individuals who had received blood transfusions from people who were later diagnosed with cancer. These donors likely had early cancers that weren't yet detected. The study looked at the recipients of these blood donations and found that they had no greater risk of developing cancer than did the general public.

The bottom line is that I can give blood. I'm still a bit needle-shy from my months of chemo, but it's good to know that my blood is welcomed.

I was also happy to learn that I'm eligible to be an organ donor.

I called the United Network for Organ Sharing, the national organization that coordinates organ donations, and learned that they encourage everyone, even sick people, to check that they are organ donors. Upon death, they'll do a variety of tests to be sure the organs are usable. Cancer does not necessarily prevent a person's organs from being used to help someone else. It's the transplant team's job to sort out what they can use and what they can't.

That was a relief. I like checking the box "I am an organ donor."

Survivors Can Help the Newly Diagnosed

People who have had cancer are often asked for advice by those who are newly diagnosed. And quite a few of us feel compelled to give our advice whether it's requested or not.

Some are these conversations are clearly beneficial to the person who's newly diagnosed, while other conversations leave them looking mostly befuddled and/or terrified.

Some general guidelines might be useful:

The most important rule for the survivor is to do more listening than talking. The conversation isn't about you—it's about the person who was just diagnosed. When someone tells that you that they were just been diagnosed with cancer, they're looking more for understanding than for advice.

The other important rule is to make the distinction between sharing your own experiences versus telling the newly diagnosed what's best for them. It's fine to say, "This is what I did," but don't say, "This is what you should do."

Keep in mind that there are more than two hundred types of cancer and they differ considerably in terms of treatment, prognosis, and impact on one's life. Your experience with thyroid cancer doesn't necessarily translate well to someone else's diagnosis with tonsil cancer. And people with the same diagnosis can have entirely different experiences. For example, there are many types of lymphoma, and there are even several different types of breast cancer. They aren't all the same.

People who are newly diagnosed tend to worry about "what if" scenarios. They ask themselves: What if the cancer has spread? What if my treatment doesn't work? What if my spouse breaks an ankle and can't drive the car to buy groceries for our family?

These thoughts aren't always rational, but they're understandable. Survivors don't need to make the newly diagnosed feel even more anxious by sharing every bad experience they've ever had or heard about.

You don't need to be irrationally positive, but you shouldn't be aggressively negative either.

And no matter how serious the diagnosis, it's important for the person to maintain hope. Not only hope for a cure, but hope for a smooth treatment process.

In sum, survivors can best help the newly diagnosed by listening and supporting. As the Shaker saying goes, "Let your words be few and seasoned with grace."

Cancer as a Chronic Disease

Until recently, people have undergone cancer treatment with the goal of ridding the body of cancer. Sometimes the treatment worked and the cancer went away, either temporarily (a remission) or permanently (a cure). If the treatment did not work, the cancer generally got worse and the person died. Success or failure.

Today, a new category of cancer care is emerging: the management of cancer as a chronic disease. Some cancers aren't curable, but they're *controllable*, with a good quality of life, for years or even decades. Many advanced or metastatic cancers fall into this category. Just as many people live with diabetes or HIV/AIDS, many people are increasingly able to live with cancer.

Living with cancer as a chronic disease is made possible, in part, by the availability of new chemotherapy drugs. In the past, only one treatment may have been available for a particular type of cancer. If that stopped working (or never worked), there were no other tools to try. Today, when Treatment A stops working, the person might be switched to Treatment B, and later to Treatment C. (You might hear this referred to as *first-line* treatment, *second-line* treatment, and so forth.)

I visit with people receiving chemotherapy almost every day. Most come for a period of three or four months, but a few come in for chemo week after week and month after month. You'd expect these "frequent fliers" to be really sick, but many look good and seem remarkably upbeat. (I'm always reminded of the television show *Cheers*. I half expect Norm to walk in and plop himself into a chemo chair as everyone calls out his name.)

People are able to tolerate long-term chemo because many of the newest drugs have fewer side effects than traditional chemotherapy drugs, and the side effects from all types of chemo are now managed better than ever before. The awful nausea that accompanied chemotherapy a generation ago is now quite rare.

I also think that people in long-term treatment become quite adept at setting priorities and managing their time. There's a rhythm to chemotherapy, and people know when they'll feel good and when they won't. The good times are reserved for what's most important and/or what's most enjoyable.

People in treatment also relish simply feeling good. When you're healthy, you take feeling good for granted. When you're sick, feeling good is a gift like the first day of spring.

Thinking of cancer as a chronic disease is new and progress in incremental. Some cancers have effective second—and third-line treatments available while others don't. And, at some point, all cancers have the ability to mutate and become resistant to every tool in the oncologist's toolbox. There is still plenty of uncertainty. But for many people with advanced cancers, a new era of treatment is emerging. The absence of a cure is not the absence of hope.

Beginning to talk about Hospice

I often talk with individuals who are receiving treatment for advanced cancer, but who are also wondering, at some level, if it's time for hospice. Many tell me that they've made the mental shift to focus on the *quality* of life rather than the *quantity* of life, but then add that they haven't contacted hospice or even discussed the possibility because "their family isn't there yet."

It is a difficult topic to discuss and that contributes to the fact that many people receive hospice care only during their final few *days* rather than their final few *months*. That's too bad because hospice is much more about living than it is about dying. When I'm ready for hospice, I want to be there long enough to enjoy the entire vacation, not just the final landing.

My advice to people is to contact their local hospice *before* they need it. I compare it to high school sophomores and juniors beginning to explore colleges. Visiting a college campus does not commit a person to attend that college or even to apply there. It just makes one familiar with the options that are available when the time is right.

Another advantage of contacting hospice early is having the opportunity to discuss those difficult end-of-life issues in the best possible setting. It's so much better to have these discussions before there's a crisis. Social workers and other hospice staff members can gently ask the right questions so that the patient's wishes are clear and heard by everyone. Again, this sets nothing in stone but it does provide a framework for making decisions when they *have* to be made at some point in the future.

Unlike hospice which is for the terminally ill (usually defined as having a life expectancy of six months or less), palliative care is available to anyone with a serious illness, without regard to life expectancy or to treatment status. (You can still be engaged in curative treatment.)

Palliative care is primarily a consultative service that focuses on symptom control and helping individuals and families communicate about end-of-life decisions. This is what they do on a daily basis and they're really good at it.

I also encourage patients to speak openly with their physicians about how long and under which conditions they wish to continue treatment. Other members of the patient's health care team are also willing to listen and provide guidance.

For example, if receiving chemotherapy, the patient might find it easier to begin having these conversations with the chemo nurses. (Chemo nurses and their patients love each other. That's just the way it is.) Bringing up the topic is better than OK, it's encouraged.

I personally want to know when hospice is a *reasonable* option, not when it becomes the *only* option. The more you communicate, the more you get what you really want.

Personal Reflections and Random Essays

My Cancer Experience

I've been writing this column for several years, and I often make passing reference to my personal experience with cancer. Today, I wanted to share my story more fully.

I first noticed a small lump under my left nipple when I was scratching my chest one summer night. I wasn't especially concerned until a few weeks later when I realized that there was blood coming out of that nipple. My first reaction was more surprise than worry. I never knew that my nipple had any plumbing behind it. I had always assumed it was more or less ornamental.

I went to see my family doctor who sent me to a surgeon who did a biopsy. The report came back, "breast cancer." I was 40 years old, in good health, had no family history of the disease, but there I was writing "mastectomy" on my calendar for August 30. It all seemed very surreal.

Although breast cancer is rare in men, it's essentially the same disease as it is in women. One difference is that men almost always undergo a mastectomy. Of course, losing a breast does not have the same significance for a man as for a woman. On the flip side, men are more likely to go around shirtless. I'm usually the only single-nippled fellow in the pool.

Chemotherapy was the scariest part of treatment because I didn't know what to expect. It was all explained to me, of course, but I didn't know how my body would react. Actually getting the chemo seemed rather anticlimactic—they put in an IV, dripped in some drugs, put on a band-aid and sent me home. I waited for bad things to happen. Fortunately, my side effects were relatively mild, with fatigue being the primary problem. I never threw up once. Ironically, my dog threw up the very first night of my chemo. I would have appreciated her empathy more had she not made a mess of the carpet.

Shortly after being diagnosed, I opened a fortune cookie and read a message that said, "You have yet to live the best years of your life." I wasn't sure if I was supposed to find that comforting or worrisome.

For the past ten years, I've worked at the Cancer Resource Center of the Finger Lakes. (Until a few years ago, we were known as the Ithaca Breast Cancer Alliance.) Most of our work involves helping people through a cancer diagnosis and treatment. Sometimes what we do is listen and give people space to think through their options. Other times, we track down information or help with such practicalities as getting to care and paying for it.

People often ask how cancer changed me. I used to focus more on long-range plans. After my diagnosis, I began to focus more on the present and the near-term. I worry less about the future and ask myself if I'm happy and if I'm making a difference in my community. The bumper sticker on my car sums up my feelings: "I'd rather be here now."

Don't Ask about My Battle

We seem to struggle with language when the topic is cancer.

We don't think twice when cancer is discussed in military terms. In 1971, Richard Nixon declared "war" on cancer in his State of the Union address.

When I was diagnosed with breast cancer, countless people told me to "fight this thing." Since I'm still alive, I'm often referred to as a survivor. If I were to die, my obituary might well read, "Bob lost his long and courageous battle with cancer."

The language of cancer seems to mirror the language of war. Battles are won and lost. There are survivors and there are victims. But is this the language we should be using?

Over the last few years, I've had several friends die from cancer. I don't think it's appropriate to say that they lost their battles. That seems to blame them for not fighting hard enough.

I prefer to say that cancer was the cause of their deaths.

In a similar fashion, I'm not quite comfortable being referred to as a survivor of cancer. Survivor is a better term than victim, but survivor seems to indicate victory. I'm not sure that I have beaten cancer. There's always the chance it might come back. (In an odd way, I'll know that I survived cancer when I die from something else.)

And what if I were living with metastatic cancer—that is, what if the cancer had spread to other parts of my body? Would I still be called a survivor? I'm not sure, but I wouldn't want anyone to think that I had lost or was losing. I would want people to think that I was living with cancer to the best of my ability.

Even the treatment for cancer is saddled with awkward language. I suspect that most people have heard chemotherapy being referred to as poison. Chemotherapy is medicine. Any medicine—even aspirin—can be poisonous if taken incorrectly. Why should chemotherapy be singled out for its potential dangers and not for its potential benefits?

Casual conversations about cancer also cause people to speak in seemingly bizarre code. I often hear people refer to cancer as the Big C. Why don't we call diabetes the Big D or eczema the Big E?

Although cancer still makes us tongue-tied, we've made real progress in that we're trying to talk about it.

Fifty years ago, people often died of cancer without ever being told the diagnosis. (Of course, most people dying of cancer knew they were dying of cancer, whether they were told or not.) And today, more and more people are living—in every sense of the word—after a cancer diagnosis.

But we still have a ways to go in being comfortable with the language of cancer.

I'll be happy to discuss my cancer with you. Just don't ask about my battle. Ask about me.

Surprising Facts about Cancer

I enjoy speaking with groups about cancer. I usually talk about my personal experiences and then describe cancer more generally and answer questions. After doing this for many years, I know that certain facts always surprise people in the audience. Here are some of those surprises:

If chemotherapy causes you to lose your hair, you'll likely lose *all* of your body hair—even the hair in your nostrils. That's why people on chemo sometimes have drippy noses. (The things we don't appreciate until there's a problem!)

If cancer metastasizes (or spreads) from one organ into another, it doesn't become a second cancer. For example, if breast cancer spreads to a person's lungs, the cancer within the lungs is not lung cancer, it's breast cancer and is treated with breast cancer drugs.

The lifetime risk for developing cancer in the United States is now one in three for women, and one in two for men.

We often talk about cancer as being one disease, but there are more than two hundred different types of cancer. They vary widely in terms of prognosis and impact on one's life. And our progress in treating each cancer varies as well—testicular cancer can now be cured even if it's relatively advanced. That's not true for most other cancers.

Significant nausea from chemotherapy is now uncommon.

Lung cancer kills many more women than breast cancer.

The five-year survival mark is not magical. Some cancers can return ten or more years later. But the risk of a recurrence goes down for each year that passes cancer-free.

The end of treatment is often as psychologically stressful as the beginning of treatment. Making the transition back to "normal" is often unexpectedly difficult and slow.

Fatigue is a nearly universal side effect of cancer treatment that people don't appreciate until it knocks them on their butts.

Cancer is increasingly thought of as a chronic disease. We used to think that people were cured of cancer or they died. Now, people are often able to *live* with cancer for many years with a good quality of life.

People often think of surgery, chemotherapy, and radiation as the three forms of cancer treatment. A fourth type of therapy—hormone therapy—can be just as important in the treatment of many types of breast, prostate, and other hormone-sensitive cancers.

Chemotherapy and/or radiation are now sometimes given *before* surgery for certain types of cancer, including breast and rectal cancers. Shrinking the tumor may reduce the scope of surgery that's required.

Uncertainty and Commitments

Being diagnosed with cancer changes one's sense of the future.

You wonder if you'll die from cancer and, if so, when.

There's rarely a definite answer to these questions, so uncertainty becomes an unwanted companion.

For the most part, this uncertainty is an abstraction floating around in the back of your head, but it becomes concrete at unexpected times.

For me, it became real when I thought about investing the money in my retirement account. Before cancer, I assumed that I would eventually enjoy many years of healthy retirement. After cancer, I wasn't so sure that I would even reach retirement age. Investing for the long-term suddenly seemed risky.

When I bought a car a few months after my surgery, I wondered if the car or I would last longer. (I'm happy to report that we're both functioning reasonably well many years later. Our bodies exhibit some dents and rust, but the engines still have some pep).

My cancer hasn't returned, and, although there's a slight risk of a recurrence, I'm again working on the assumption that I'll enjoy many years of retirement.

But other people with cancer aren't so fortunate.

A woman in treatment asked me a blunt question: "How can I make commitments when I'm dealing with a crappy diagnosis?"

She went on, "It's hard for me to commit to doing something next week because I don't know how I'll feel. And bigger commitments—like starting a new relationship or a new job—seem impossible."

She was asking the question rhetorically, but I've been thinking about it ever since.

I wish I had a simple answer.

I do know that living with uncertainty is easier if you're surrounded by people who understand and accept that uncertainty. They are there for you no matter what.

It's so much more difficult without that support.

As we enter the holiday season, we tend to think about life in the bigger picture. Where we are, where we are headed, and who we are with.

Serious illness adds poignancy and even urgency to these thoughts.

At a recent cancer support group, Rev. Tim Dean, Chaplain at Cayuga Medical Center, said that serious illness often makes us more authentic.

Perhaps that's why making commitments is sometimes more difficult when cancer is present. The commitments need to be honest and authentic. There's not much pretense when you're bald from chemotherapy.

But perhaps that is some of the good that can emerge from the bad of cancer. When someone is with you through cancer, or even after cancer, they are with you all the way.

The Ugly Stepsister of Cancer

There's a warm and fuzzy side to breast cancer. Not the disease itself, which is life-disruptive at its best and deadly at its worst. But there are celebratory races with survivors crossing the finish line with arms raised in triumph, magazine covers honoring celebrities who have survived the disease, and pink ribbons seemingly everywhere.

Other cancers receive less attention. These cancers may not have a warm and fuzzy side, but we agree that people diagnosed with them deserve our support and kindness.

But one cancer is noteworthy for the lack of empathy and compassion it elicits.

"Lung cancer is the ugly stepsister of cancer," was how one person described it to me.

When she was diagnosed, most people assumed that she smoked. She didn't. (Some ten to fifteen percent of people diagnosed with lung cancer are nonsmokers. For reasons not fully understood, lung cancer is more common in nonsmoking women than in nonsmoking men.)

Even her friends who knew she didn't smoke interrogated her to find the cause. There was an underlying sense that if she wasn't at fault, someone or something else was.

This seems to be a common theme with lung cancer. Blame is the elephant in the room. People with other cancers aren't blamed. We don't accuse them or even wonder if they did something to cause their cancers. The cancer just is.

Anyone who has had cancer can tell you how difficult it was to get the diagnosis and then to share that news with family and friends. Imagine how much more difficult it would be if you sensed people thinking—or even saying—"Well, that's what you get for smoking."

And, assuming that an individual did smoke, what difference does that make once they have lung cancer? Should we be less compassionate or less supportive? Absolutely not.

I'm hardly an apologist for smokers or for the tobacco industry. I hate it when smokers foul my air and increase my insurance rates. I make it a point not to enter a business if I see employees smoking near its front door. And I want to shake sense into young people when I see them lighting up.

But if you have lung cancer, you don't need blame. You need kindness and support, given without judgment.

Cancer and the Nature of Hope

Cancer and hope are two topics that often intersect.

People with cancer sometimes wonder if maintaining hope in the face of a grim diagnosis is a good idea or a bad idea.

My response is that hope is always good, but it's a mistake to define hope strictly in the context of being cured.

When a person is first diagnosed with cancer, hope and cure do overlap. People hope that they will be cured. Even if the survival rate cancer is only ten percent, somebody has to be in that ten percent and it might as well be you.

Or it might be said, "People with your cancer can expect to live about twelve months." What that means is that half of the people with your cancer will live longer than twelve months.

Statistics provide guideposts, but they don't dictate what will happen to a specific individual.

Of course, cancer can metastasize or otherwise advance to the point that a cure is unrealistic.

But does this mean giving up hope? No, not at all. But it does mean reframing your concept of hope to something other than a cure.

Many people who can't be cured can hope for months or years of continuing to live with a good quality of life.

Even people with a terminal diagnosis can and should have hope. The hope may be as modest as having a good weekend or as significant as a reconciliation with an estranged family member.

Hope is somehow at the core of our being human, even when one's current situation is difficult. Thich Nhat Hanh wrote, "Hope is important because it can make the present moment less difficult to bear. If we believe that tomorrow will be better, we can bear a hardship today."

And there is the hope that our lives have had and will continue to have meaning.

Hope is always present.

I have cancer. What's new with you?

Two days after being diagnosed with cancer, I received a call from the Red Cross asking if I'd give blood in an upcoming blood drive.

I was a regular blood donor, so I received these calls a couple of times a year.

This time, my head nearly exploded with a thousand thoughts: Should I tell this anonymous person that I have cancer? Will she write "Bob Riter has cancer" in some computerized database? Can people with cancer give blood?

I said, "Sorry, I can't make it this time."

When I hung up, I realized that I had been unable to say, "I can't give blood because I was just diagnosed with cancer."

The words "I have cancer" seemed to get stuck in my throat.

Nearly everyone who gets diagnosed with cancer struggles saying those words at first. It's an admission that you really do have cancer and that much in life is suddenly so different.

The first people you tell are your family and close friends. That's emotional, but you know that they're somehow in this journey with you.

Telling more casual acquaintances can be downright weird. People often ask, "How are you?" as a form of greeting. They expect to hear, "Fine. Yourself?"

A new cancer diagnosis makes "how are you?" a difficult question.

For weeks, I wrestled with what to say to whom. I'd ask myself, "How well do I know this person? Who are their friends and who will they tell? Will their feelings be hurt if I don't tell them?"

No wonder shopping at the supermarket was exhausting. I had too many mental calculations to make when people asked, "Hi Bob. What's up with you?"

I once responded to "how are you?" by saying, "Well, I was just diagnosed with breast cancer and I'm going to have a mastectomy next week and then a few months of chemotherapy. What's new with you?"

Although his expression was priceless, I decided that wasn't the smoothest approach.

As time went by, I became more relaxed about talking about my cancer. Nearly everyone was supportive, and many people stepped up and became dearer friends than ever before.

I did lose a few acquaintances. For whatever reason, they couldn't handle my having cancer and they gradually disappeared from my life. I think they weren't sure what to say at first and later felt awkward about never having said anything. (By the way, it's never too late to reconnect with those who have been ill. A card that says, "My thoughts continue to be with you" are always welcomed.)

It's now many years after my cancer diagnosis, and I'm about as open about my cancer as one can be. I'm not above showing my mastectomy scar to total strangers over dinner.

But I still remember how difficult it was for me to say, "I have cancer," when the Red Cross called that night.

My *Cancer Sucks* Button

I often wear a button that says *cancer sucks*. In addition to pretty well summing up the cancer experience, it's a great conversation starter.

Just last month, a man tapped my button as I was waiting in line for coffee in the San Antonio airport. He nodded sadly and told me that his young daughter was being treated for cancer in Houston. Since the button seemed to strike a chord with him, I asked if he'd like to have it. At first he shook his head, but I assured him that I had more in my office. He took it from me, attached it to his coat, and left to catch his flight.

It was one of those fleeting moments of shared humanity. We talked for only a few seconds, but the connection was real.

That's the thing about cancer. It allows us to connect with others by a kind of shorthand that cuts across the usual boundaries of gender, race, age, and class.

When I meet someone with cancer, or affected by cancer, I have a fairly good idea of what they're experiencing.

But it's important to realize that I don't know *exactly* what they're experiencing. Every cancer is different and every individual is different. This was brought home recently when a woman affected by a head and neck cancer told me, "I envy you people with breast cancer because you can put on your shirt and cover your scars."

That gave me pause.

Cancer can bring people together for another reason as well: it's a great equalizer.

An acquaintance was reading about a celebrity diagnosed with cancer and said she didn't have much sympathy for him because he had the money and connections to get the best possible care.

My reaction was quite different. When you're diagnosed with cancer, you're scared no matter how famous you are or how much money you have.

That's one of the reasons I wear my button. Cancer is scary, but it's a little less scary if we talk about it.

Small Acts of Heroism

TV shows and magazine articles routinely recognize heroes at this time of year. In keeping with that theme, I thought I would select an individual who's been especially heroic in the face of cancer and write an inspirational holiday column about him or her. But the more I thought about it, the more I realized that heroism in the cancer world—the world I inhabit—isn't the heroism that we see in the movies. It's far more nuanced and, well, real. What I see are daily acts of courage that occur without fanfare, but deserve to be noticed.

Simply beginning cancer treatment is a courageous act. Surgery, chemotherapy, and radiation therapy are scary for everyone. I often hear people say afterward, "I never thought I could do it, but I did."

Although not speaking specifically about cancer, Eleanor Roosevelt captured this feeling: "You gain strength, courage, and confidence by every experience in which you really stop to look fear in the face. *You must do the thing which you think you cannot do.*"

Here are examples of the courage I see:

> There was a young man who decided to quit smoking just as he began chemotherapy. At an age when it's easy to stick one's head in the sand or blame everyone else, he acknowledged his problems and dealt with them.

> There was the woman who managed to keep working during months of difficult chemotherapy by adapting her work schedule to the rhythms of the treatment.

There was a man with mental illness who underwent treatment with remarkable dignity and courage.

There was the guy who hated hospitals and doctors, but came with his wife to support her quietly through every one of her appointments and treatments.

There were the women who crowded the hospital room of a colleague who was just diagnosed with cancer. No one knew quite what to say, but they knew that being there was important.

There was the man who stepped in and helped his older brother feel connected and supported during his final months.

There was the couple that were so loving towards each other and so gracious to everyone else in the chemo suite that they made us all better by just being near.

Time and time again, I see cancer bring out the best in people. Maybe we're at our best when we deal with what's real and cancer certainly is just that. Robert Frost put it like this: "The best way out is always through." People do their best to get through their treatment, through their illness, or simply through their day. Heroism is everywhere in the people I see. It's the small and seemingly simple acts of courage that constantly amaze and inspire me. We should all take note of the people whose lives have been touched by cancer and recognize the courage they have shown by doing what they thought they could not do.

The Uncertainty of Cancer

Before you get diagnosed with cancer, you assume that it will be an unpleasant experience, but one that is pretty straightforward.

One might think, "I have this type of cancer, so I will get that type of treatment." Like getting a hernia fixed, only more serious. But cancer is filled with uncertainty, and hardly anyone is prepared for it.

Patients often ask: Why did I get cancer? Will I be cured? Which side effects will I experience? Which treatment is best?

Oncologists often respond to these questions by saying, "I don't know." They aren't hiding anything—they really don't know. No one does.

Uncertainty can occur because there's so much variation in how individuals respond to treatment.

You can give two people the exact same chemotherapy drugs—one will sail through without any problems and the other will feel awful every single day.

One person will be cured by a particular treatment and another individual with the same diagnosis will have a recurrence within a few months.

Sometimes uncertainty exists because there's no data that specifically answers the question. For example, I'm a guy with breast cancer. There isn't much research on treating male breast cancer, so it's generally assumed that what works for post-menopausal women will work for me, too.

Entirely reasonable, but not altogether reassuring.

Even common cancers are fraught with uncertainty. Men with prostate cancer may be given the options of surgery, radiation, or watchful waiting. Sometimes the best option for a particular patient is clear. Other times, it's a complete toss-up.

Uncertainty continues after treatment is completed. The big question for most people is whether the cancer will return.

As someone who has had cancer, let me say that this uncertainty really sucks.

But a change in perspective can be positive as well.

I was walking my dog on a cloudy Ithaca day when she came across a ray of sunlight hitting the sidewalk. She immediately sat down, closed her eyes and relished the pure joy of sitting in the sun. That image of her living purely in the moment stays with me. And my cancer, as cancers go, was pretty good. That is, my risk of a recurrence is low, especially now that several years have passed. But I no longer feel invincible. Of course, you don't have to have cancer to face uncertainty. It's part of the human experience.

Several people have said to me, "Too bad you got cancer, but life is uncertain for everyone. I could be hit by a bus tomorrow." (I'm never sure how to respond to this comment. "God willing" seems a bit awkward.)

Cancer and uncertainty do go hand-in-hand. It's good in some ways and bad in others. Like many other realities, it just is and we go forward the best we can.

The Difficult Transitions of Cancer

My job is to listen to people affected by cancer and to help them however I can. With experience, I've come to understand that the periods of greatest stress and emotional turmoil are often predictable. When people come to my office, they're usually at one of four periods of critical transition.

The first critical transition is the short time between being diagnosed with cancer and beginning treatment. People have to wrap their heads around a potentially life-threatening illness, and they're typically overwhelmed with information and advice. They need to decide which treatment, if any, to pursue and are wondering if they should get a second or third opinion. Critical decisions have to be made when no one can say for sure which decision will turn out to be the "correct" one. High levels of stress during this phase are common. I reassure people that their anxiety level will go down once decisions are made and treatment is started.

The second critical transition is at the end of treatment. This seems counterintuitive, but most people are scared when they complete their last radiation therapy or chemo session. It's often described as leaving the safety of the cocoon. People miss seeing their health professionals on a regular basis, and they worry about the cancer returning. One's imagination goes into overdrive. A headache isn't just a headache, it's a brain tumor. And it takes more time than expected to bounce back and resume one's previous life. I reassure people that a post-treatment funk is both common and temporary.

The first two transitions are almost universal. The next two occur only if cancer returns.

The third critical transition is at the time of a recurrence. When cancer returns, the focus of treatment generally shifts from *curing* the cancer to *controlling* the cancer. That's a huge mental adjustment. As a friend recently said to me, "When I was first diagnosed with cancer, it was a bump in the road in my life. Now, I have advanced cancer and it *is* the road in my life." At this point, I reassure people that cancer is increasingly thought of as a chronic disease and that many are able to live, with treatment, for many years while experiencing a good quality of life.

The fourth critical transition occurs when people with advanced cancer get worse. They have to decide if they want to keep trying new treatments with the hope of living longer, or if they'd rather stop active treatment and focus on comfort and quality of life through hospice. Here, I reassure people that *they* are in control of this decision.

Living with cancer is never a straight line, but these four critical periods of transition are the times of greatest anxiety and uncertainty. If people with cancer anticipate these periods, perhaps the transitions will be a little less difficult. And if their loved ones are aware of the transitions, perhaps they will know when to be most available, most attentive, and most supportive.

The Good That Emerged

A friend with cancer wrote me to say how she now experiences moments of intense appreciation.

Just walking her dog at Buttermilk State Park filled her with tears. Not tears of sadness, but tears of unabashed appreciation of that gorgeous moment.

The dog, the forest, the beauty. They made her cry.

She said that she never had such intense feelings before her cancer.

Her comments got me to thinking that good often emerges from serious illness.

I asked the attendees at a recent cancer support group if anything positive came out of their disease. To a person, they said yes.

One woman waved her hand around the table and said that she found a remarkable sense of community with others who also have cancer. "We're in the same boat—we understand each other." She added softly, "I love that."

Another person said that cancer builds community because it's a great equalizer. "It doesn't matter if you're black or white, rich or poor, man or woman. We're all sick and we're all scared. I don't know the name of the person who's getting chemo in the chair next to me, but he's like a brother to me now."

Other people at the support group saw cancer as a personal challenge. One guy said, "Cancer is the scariest thing I've ever faced. But I found that I had the strength to get through it. I didn't think I could, but I did and I'm proud of that."

Nearly everyone expressed gratitude that they no longer take anything for granted. "I give thanks every day," said a woman, accompanied by nods from all around the table.

Trust and faith were two recurring themes. So much about cancer is uncertain that one has to plunge forward even though no one knows for certain what will happen. "Trust is hard for me, but I had to trust my doctors," said one man. "And once I gave that trust, I began to relax a little."

Many also described a renewed sense of spirituality when confronted with cancer. Faith often provides comfort during our most difficult times.

I'm often reminded of the book *Why Bad Things Happen to Good People*. Harold Kushner, the author, concluded by saying that the more important question is how people respond when bad things inevitably happen.

I'm so often impressed by how people respond to cancer with dignity, strength, and grace. Cancer isn't good and I wouldn't wish it on anyone. But only a person touched by serious illness could have written, "I was suddenly overwhelmed at how lucky I was to be alive; I was experiencing this sunny day in the forest with my beloved puppy and I started crying because it was so gorgeous."

The Look People Give You

I love it when people suggest column ideas.

I was walking through the chemo suite yesterday and a person called me over and said, "I wish you would write a column to tell people not to give me *that* look."

"What look?" I asked.

"The pity puss." (At first I thought she said "platypus" which I faintly recalled as being a weird looking animal. I wondered why on earth people were making platypus faces at her.)

Noting my momentary confusion, she continued, "Pity puss. Once I got diagnosed with cancer, people started looking at me as though I was a completely different person."

I knew the look she was referring to. When I was diagnosed, people would look at me with solemn expressions and tilted heads as if they were looking deep into my soul. That look was always unsettling, especially when I was trying to eat lunch.

I decided to play investigative reporter by asking other people with cancer if they've seen that look.

One woman told me that she knows the look, but it doesn't bother her because she knows it's coming from a place of caring. "Of course we have a list of things we want people to say or do, but cancer is emotionally loaded and scary. The solemn faces, teary eyeballs, and spiels about being brave aren't perfect gestures, but they show concern."

Another told me that she also knows the look, but what bothers her even more is the non-look. "Some people who used to make eye contact with me when saying 'good morning' now avert their eyes and hurry away fearing that a conversation might take place."

Once you've had cancer, you don't give "that look" when meeting someone else with cancer. One nurse told me, "It's like you guys with cancer have your own secret society." She's right. That's why spending time with others with cancer can be relaxing because cancer isn't an elephant in the room. If people want to talk about cancer, fine. If people don't want to talk about cancer, that's fine too.

I'm afraid that I may be making readers so paranoid of making the wrong face or saying the wrong thing that their heads might explode when encountering someone with cancer. Don't worry. What's in your heart is far more important than what you say or the expression on your face.

The most important lesson is to remember that your friend who now has cancer is the same person she was before she had cancer. If she liked hugs before, she'll like them now. If she was a private person before, she'll be a private person now.

If you're not sure what to say when you first talk with her after she's been diagnosed, try, "I'm so sorry." It's simple, honest, and so human.

Stepping Up for Neighbors

Not everyone with cancer has built-in support. Perhaps the individual has no family, or an event in the past may have caused the family to become estranged. Some people are just loners by nature and have happily kept to themselves through the years. Others are isolated because of mental illness. And some people have burned every bridge that once brought them connection.

I'd like to recognize a small group of people who step up to support a neighbor, a community member, or an acquaintance who would otherwise go through cancer alone.

This support takes many forms. Sometimes it's driving the person to treatment, bringing over a bowl of soup, or helping sort through the stack of bills on the kitchen table. Often, the most important role is to listen as the person comes to grips with having a life-threatening illness.

But I have also seen this support evolve such that the neighbor is the one who helps the patient navigate their final months of life. The neighbor becomes the de facto family—making sure that the patient is loved and that their wishes are carried out. I've even seen neighbors arrange funerals and scatter the individual's ashes afterward.

I don't think we have a word for all of this, but I wish we did. "Saintly" doesn't really work because not all of these caregivers are, well, saintly. More often, they're just normal folk who go to work, drink beer on the weekend, and try to do what's right.

They don't consciously decide to help their neighbor through their final days—it just happens. I suspect they sometimes think, "I really don't want to do this."

But they do.

I often wonder how and why people are able to help their neighbors in this way. It's certainly not done for the recognition or for money. I do believe that most people want to find meaning in life. Helping someone through illness and death—especially someone you have no obligation to help—has to be one of life's most meaningful experiences.

And, as we get older and wiser, many realize that helping a neighbor is how we best save the world.

By the very nature of what they do, these good neighbors are the last ones to leave the funeral home. There's no one left behind to thank them.

If one of you is reading this column, know that I thank you. And know that your community is a better place because of you.

New Year's Wishes

At New Year's, we're supposed to make resolutions to change our own behavior in the months to come. I think it's more fun to wave a magic wand and change the behavior of everyone else. Here's what I wish for:

I wish that people with cancer weren't beaten over the head with the importance of positive thinking.

I wish that people with lung cancer didn't get blamed for their cancer.

I wish that receptionists in every doctor's office smiled and made eye contact with everyone.

I wish that more family members asked the patient what the patient wanted and didn't assume what the patient wanted.

I wish that new cancer drugs producing modest benefits weren't marketed as major breakthroughs with exorbitant prices.

I wish that all journal articles emerging from medical research funded by the government were made available online, without charge, to the public.

I wish that exercise and nutrition received more attention in cancer prevention, treatment, and recovery.

I wish that people dealing with cancer didn't have to worry about how to pay for it.

I wish that the relatives, friends and neighbors of people newly diagnosed with cancer refrained from giving advice (except when requested).

I wish that the prevention of cancer received the same attention and funding as the diagnosis and treatment of cancer.

I wish that everyone with cancer took the time to thank their loved ones for always being there.

I wish that people didn't assume that the most aggressive cancer treatment was always the best cancer treatment.

I wish that every cancer patient understood that reality and hope aren't mutually exclusive.

I don't have a magic wand, but I will keep wishing.

Our Cancer Professionals

I often write about the resilience and grace of people who have cancer. Today, I'd like to shine a light on the doctors, nurses, and therapists who provide their care.

I suspect most people—and many health professionals—think of treating cancer patients as being depressing. It's not. But it is challenging. Some of those challenges are fairly obvious—people with cancer are often very sick, death sometimes looms as a possible outcome, and everyone in the waiting room is scared.

Other challenges are less obvious. A cancer diagnosis affects the entire family. Family members have questions and opinions, and family dynamics (both good and bad) are amplified. It's not unusual for the patient to be the calmest person in the room.

Treating cancer patients requires what I think of as compartmentalization. The professional has to be completely present with each patient and not thinking about the previous patient or the next one. This is a skill that doesn't come naturally to most of us. This is especially difficult in oncology because some patients are doing great, some are dying, and others are living in a world of uncertainty. The gamut of human emotions can be witnessed in a single morning.

Another challenge is responding to questions that don't have definitive answers. Patients often want to know what the future holds for them. Statistics can provide general guides, but no one knows for sure how an individual will respond to a particular treatment or if their cancer will return. By its very nature, cancer is unpredictable.

Science is the starting point of cancer care, but there is an art to applying that science to each patient. This art is based on clinical experience, judgment, and intuition. Patients don't always fit into neat little boxes with obvious choices for the best treatment.

The importance of communication can't be overstated. Patients need to understand their treatment options and the probable benefits and risks of pursuing those options. Try explaining anything to people of differing ages, education levels, and cultural values. Then try it when those people are scared and part of what needs to be explained is uncertain. It isn't easy.

I want to make special mention of chemotherapy nurses and radiation therapists who work with cancer patients throughout the course of treatment. In addition to providing care, they often become the grounding force that keeps the patient together during these difficult months. Something as simple as a calming hand on the shoulder can make a remarkable difference. Sometimes the patients use the nurses and therapists as relief valves—patients can say things that they can't say to their family members. In some ways, the therapy room is a safe place because the word "cancer" doesn't make anyone flinch.

I said earlier that working with cancer patients isn't depressing, but there are inevitable times of sadness. People die, sometimes unexpectedly so. And there are also times of happiness when people do well and return to their lives, cured of what was once an incurable disease.

What I've come to realize is that there is always something that can be done to help a person with cancer. Even if the disease can't be cured, a patient's quality of life can be affected in a positive manner. It's not a profession for everyone. But I'm happy that so many good people have chosen it.

New Nurses and Cancer Patients

Most everyone is uncertain and tentative when first talking with people who are in treatment for cancer. What should you say? What should you not say?

This is just as true for health professionals as it is for members of the general public. Even hospital employees sometimes feel tongue-tied when cancer is the diagnosis.

I recently spoke with a class of nursing students at Tompkins Cortland Community College. One woman raised her hand and said, "I'll soon graduate and begin working in a hospital. What should I do to help my patients who have cancer?"

I thought it was a great question, and I've since asked several experienced oncology nurses what they would have shared with the students. This is what they said:

> Don't be afraid of silence. Sometimes you can best support patients by simply being with them without talking.

> Don't reflexively say, "Everything will be fine," or some other reassuring sentiment. It's better to ask, "How are you doing with all of this?"

> Don't assume that what you would want is what they should want. Don't even think, let alone say, "You'd be crazy not to have this treatment. It will extend your life."

> Be vigilant about pain control. If the patient is in pain, call the doctor. If the patient continues to be in pain, call the doctor again.

Gently remind patients that they—not their family members or even their doctors—are in charge of treatment decisions.

Listen to the patients, especially those who have had cancer for a while. They know much more about their cancer than you do.

Ask the patient to tell you their story in their own words. You'll learn about their cancer and about them.

Be aware of the patient's social situation. Is there support at home? Is the patient likely to fall between the cracks and not receive care after leaving the hospital?

Understand that cancer affects the entire family. Loved ones are often more stressed than the person with cancer.

Use each patient as a learning experience—study their specific type of cancer. What you learn will stay with you because you have a face to go with that diagnosis.

Be aware of support programs within the hospital (e.g., the chaplain) and in the community (e.g., cancer support organizations) and suggest them to patients when appropriate.

If you have questions, contact the hospital's oncology nurses. They're usually happy to talk about their work and share their knowledge with you.

Several of the nurses I talked with said that they never expected to work in oncology, but they do and they love it. One put it this way, "I once thought cancer was about death and dying, but it's not. It's all about life and living."

Doing What I Do

I often talk with people while they're receiving chemotherapy. Recently, one woman asked, "How long have you been doing this?"

I knew that she was talking about my work, so I replied that I've been visiting with cancer patients for more than ten years. She then asked, "How do you do it?"

She went on, "You deal with cancer every single day. Some patients won't ever get better. And nearly everyone you talk with must be scared, sick, or both.

Doesn't it depress the hell out of you?"

I've been reflecting on this question ever since.

Although the question was directed to me, it just as easily could have been directed to the doctors, nurses, radiation therapists, and others who work with cancer patients on a regular basis.

I posed the question to a nurse who responded, "Everyone who begins cancer treatment will have an outcome. Sometimes that outcome is a cure, sometimes it's not a cure, but a longer life, and sometimes the outcome is that the person dies no matter what we do."

She said, "I can't focus on the outcomes—I focus on the journey. I can make the journey better for people and doing so brings me satisfaction."

One physician told me she wishes that no one would ever say the words, "There's nothing we can do." She said, "There's *always* something we can do. We can control pain, we can provide comfort, we can listen."

A hospital chaplain told me that his job is to be with people when they're in dark and scary places. It's not a matter of fixing what sometimes can't be fixed. It's a matter of sharing the experience so that no one is alone.

There's an underlying theme to all of these comments. Working with people with cancer requires a focus on what you can do, rather than on what you cannot do.

The losses that inevitably occur in oncology affect everyone who shares that space and that journey. It's essential to have loved ones and coworkers who understand and provide nurturing.

We're also bolstered by those patients and their family members who come in and somehow make life better for everyone in the room. Some possess a quiet dignity and some crack goofy jokes that make us laugh.

There's a lot of love in the chemo suite and in radiation medicine.

And don't forget that many people diagnosed with cancer are cured and go on to live rich, full lives. I often see former patients—who were once bald and pale—looking the picture of health.

But it's also good to see the patients who aren't doing do so well. We may not know what's ahead, but it's a privilege to share in that journey.

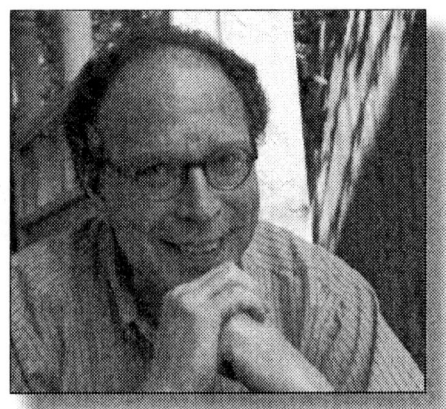

Bob Riter is the Executive Director of the Cancer Resource Center of the Finger Lakes, an organization that provides support, information and community to people affected by cancer in and around Ithaca, NY. In addition, Bob writes a regular column about living with cancer for the Ithaca Journal. Those columns serve as the foundation for this book.

Bob's involvement with cancer support and education began in 1996 when he was diagnosed with breast cancer. A native of Huntington, WV, Bob received his undergraduate degree from Oberlin College and a master's degree in health services administration from the University of Michigan.

The proceeds from the sale of this book go to the
Cancer Resource Center to further its work and support
its belief that no one should face cancer alone.